SOMATIC EXERCISES FOR BEGINNERS

The Complete Guide To Weight Loss, Stress Relief And Emotional Well-Being

Merton Corey

Copyright:

© 2023 Merton Corey. All rights reserved. No part of this publication may be reproduced, distributed, or transmitted in any form or by any means, including photocopying, recording, or other electronic or mechanical methods, without the prior written permission of the publisher, except in the case of brief quotations embodied in critical reviews and certain other noncommercial uses permitted by copyright law.

Disclaimer:

The information provided in this book is intended for general informational and educational purposes only. The author is not a licensed medical professional, and the content in this book should not be considered a substitute for professional medical advice, diagnosis, or treatment. Always seek the advice of your physician or qualified healthcare provider before beginning any fitness program or making significant changes to your diet or exercise routine.

The author and publisher have made reasonable efforts to ensure that the information presented in this book is accurate and reliable at the time of publication. However, they do not warrant the completeness, reliability, or accuracy of this information. The author and publisher disclaim any liability for any adverse effects or consequences resulting from the use of the information contained herein, either directly or indirectly.

By reading this book, you acknowledge and agree that you are solely responsible for any actions you take based on the information provided, and you release the author and the publisher from any liability for any damages or injuries, whether direct or indirect, that may result.

TABLE OF CONTENTS

INTRODUCTION 4
   BENEFITS OF SOMATIC EXERCISES: 4
   KEY TIPS ON HOW TO PERFORM THE EXERCISES 6
HOW TO READ THE BOOK FOR MAXIMAL RESULTS: 7
EXERCISES 9
   FLOOR STAR 9
   BABY STRETCH 11
   PELVIC PREPARATION 13
   EAGLE POSE 15
   MOVING ROCK 17
   NECK AND HIPS 19
   CHEST OPENING 21
   DESPAIR 23
   ROLL IN 25
   ROLL OUT 27
   SUPERMAN 29
   SIDE REACH 31
   SPINAL WAVE 33
   REACH BACK 35
   STANDING REACH 37
   SPIDER CIRCLE 39
   STAR GLUTE BRIDGE 41
   STANDING STRESS RELEASE 43
   STANDING SPIDER 45
   FULL BODY ROCKING 47
   STRETCH AND COMPRESS 49
   ENERGY OPENING 51
   KNEE HOLD 53
   NECK RELEASE 55
   OPEN LIFE 57
   JUMPING JACKS 59
   BURPEES 61
   FLOWER 63
   OPEN UP PLANK 65
28-DAY PLAN 67
CONCLUSION 83

INTRODUCTION

Somatic exercises are a practice that can be done anywhere; all you need is a bit of space and a mat. Therefore, it does not require specific requirements or expensive tools. The main difference between somatic exercises and others is that somatic exercise is more like a sensory experience. It focuses on how you feel while performing the exercise and aims to address and release negative sensations - just a few daily minutes consistently can bring you the results you desire.

Somatic exercises primarily aim to resolve trauma, pain, and tension through relatively easy and fluid movements. In this book, the exercises have been studied not only to achieve these goals but also to improve a person's fitness by enhancing flexibility and their connection with their body. Each exercise is instructed step by step as well as explaining the benefits for doing each one of them

This book is not simply a list of exercises to do; it's important to emphasize that focusing on the internal experience and feelings while practicing is key. The majority of the exercises are 'Grounding Exercises' that help you feel connected to the earth, aiding in restoring good energy and maintaining a high vibration. Ideally doing this outside on a mat works fantastically. However, if it's cold outside and/or you don't have easy access to a quiet place outside your house, feel free to do the exercises indoors (as shown in the book).

BENEFITS OF SOMATIC EXERCISES:

- **Reduce stress**

Doing consistently the routines that will be presented in the book will help drastically reduce worry and anxiety. There are many case studies where people just after 7 days of training, experience less or no anxiety.

- **Aid Weight loss**

Somatic exercises are great not only for releasing trauma and stress but also for helping weight loss. Those exercises itself will not make you lose weight but they will help you enhance metabolism by lowering your stress levels and making your muscles leaner and more toned.

Following a healthy diet and being in a caloric deficit is also tremendously important for weight loss.

- **Improve relaxation body and mind relaxation**

There are many tailored exercises that aim to release tension. This not only will make you feel more calm but also it will improve posture and body alignment.

- **Managing negative emotions effectively**

Helps to let go of: anger, despair, and discouragement that might happen during your daily life activities.

- **Increase mindfulness**

Somatic exercises will help you feel present and increase body awareness, enhancing mind-body connection as each exercise requires you to focus on your body movement as well as deep relaxation.

- **Increase flexibility**

This is a bonus that it will come after 7-14 days of doing the exercises, especially in the low back and hip area. It will release the overall tightness, leaving you feeling good and more energetic.

KEY TIPS ON HOW TO PERFORM THE EXERCISES

This book will show you in detail several exercises to maximize their benefit and help you become the best version of yourself.

So, how do you perform these movements? Since the initial aim of somatic practices is to resolve trauma and tension, it's important to focus on releasing negative feelings. Therefore, it is suggested to:

- *Focus on feelings*; it's a mindful practice centered around how you feel. As mentioned in the introduction, the distinction between somatic training and other practices lies in its formation through sensory exercises; it's not 'just' movement.

- *Start the session with a specific aim*; it can be to 'Release stress,' 'Release tension,' 'Release Anxiety,' or any other goal you have in mind. Keep in mind that regardless of your specific aim, the practice will benefit you in many ways. However, it's important to have a specific aim in mind to prepare for the exercise with the right approach. Based on my experience, people that approach these exercises with a specific goal in mind tend to stick to the exercises consistently, therefore having more results.

- *Relax your body*; regardless of your specific aim, relaxing muscles, joints, and the mind is the necessary ingredient to witness transformation in your physical and mental health.

HOW TO READ THE BOOK FOR MAXIMAL RESULTS:

As you finish the introduction, which explains what somatic exercises are, their benefits, and how to perform them. You will now move to the section on exercises, followed by the training plan.

The exercise section comprises exercises with step-by-step pictures and detailed explanations on how to perform each one. Within these pages, you'll find everything you need to know about every single exercise. At the end of each exercise, you'll notice that the duration of certain positions or the number of repetitions and sets is not specified. You will find this information in the following section. Each day will require you to perform exercises differently from the previous ones, and the plan is structured to increase the number of repetitions and sets as you progress.

In the last section, you'll discover the 28-day training plan. Follow each day diligently, don't skip workouts, maintain consistency, and adhere strictly to the daily plan. Guaranteed results will follow!

Hey! Before we start with the Somatic exercises and the 28-Day Plan

If you have any doubts, questions or simply you like to give a feedback, feel free to send an email at **mertoncoreyfitness@gmail.com**

I'll be happy to help you maximize your results!

EXERCISES

FLOOR STAR

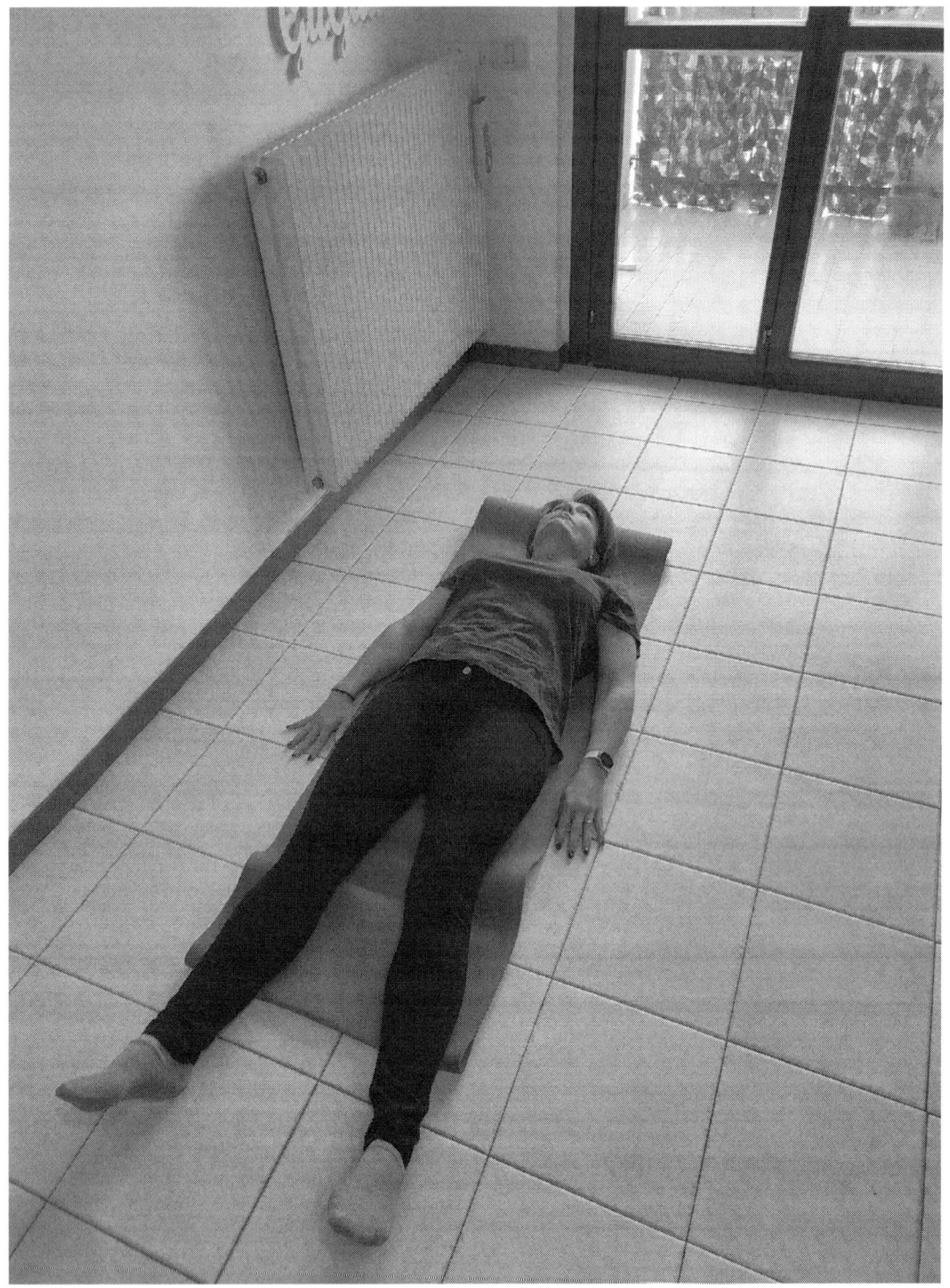

Focus on the breathing and body scan.

Benefits:

This exercise is vital for preparing for the actual session. It's important to feel relaxed and establish a connection with your body. Focus on breathing deeply and relaxing any areas that feel tight or tense. This exercise should initiate every session and should be practiced for at least 10 deep breaths. Let go of any thoughts and worry. This exercise must be done at the beginning of every session.
(It will be mentioned in the section of the 28-Day Plan too.)

How to do it:

- Lie on your back with your legs spread wider than shoulder width apart, and your arms on the side of your body.
- Concentrate on your breath, relax your body and be present in the moment.
- Pay attention to the parts touching the mat, noticing any tension or tightness. Be aware of the curve of your spine. Notice your legs and find the most comfortable position for your feet.
- Inhale through your nose and exhale through your mouth deeply at least 10 times. If you feel particularly tense, feel free to extend this exercise for a longer duration.

BABY STRETCH

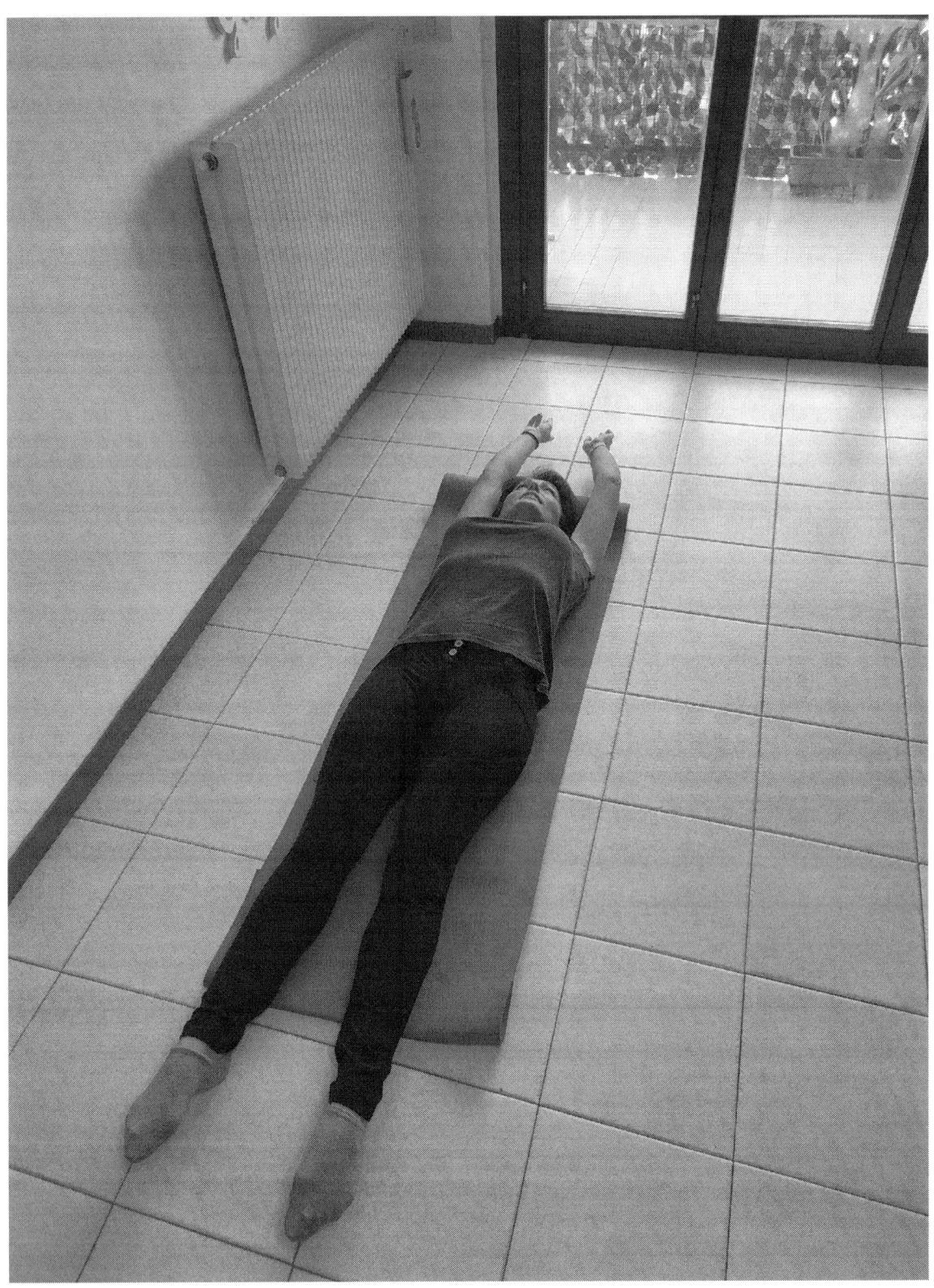

Stretch your legs and arms for mentioned reps.

Benefits:

Great exercise to extend your body and release all the tightness that you feel. The stress and trauma we have experienced tend to tighten our muscles. By doing this exercise, you release those negative emotions and gain energy. It is the most basic exercise that even babies do. It is extremely natural, or at least it should feel that way. If it does not feel comfortable or natural, it means that this exercise will massively help you to release those negative emotions. Overtime, you'll feel at ease doing it. Lastly, It also helps to improve posture and alignment of your body.

How to do it:

- Lie on your back, legs spread wider than shoulder width apart, and arms straight next to your body - just to start.
- Then, reach over your head and stretch, as shown in the image. At the same time, stretch your legs and your feet as if you are reaching for something. Feel a complete stretch in your body, like a baby after waking up. Keep the position for around 5 seconds.
- Return to the starting position, releasing the stretch, and repeat the exercise for the mentioned times.

PELVIC PREPARATION

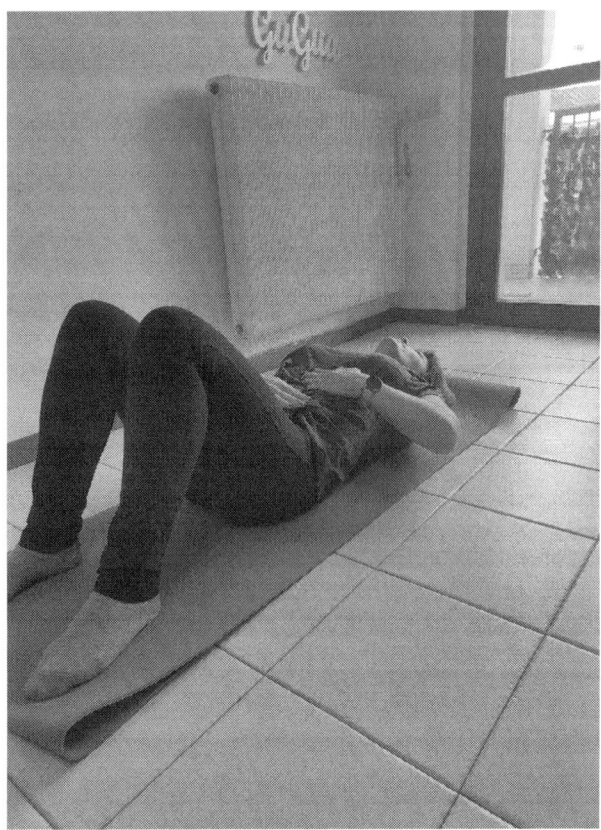

Step 1 - Squeeze your low back on the floor, and exhale through your mouth.

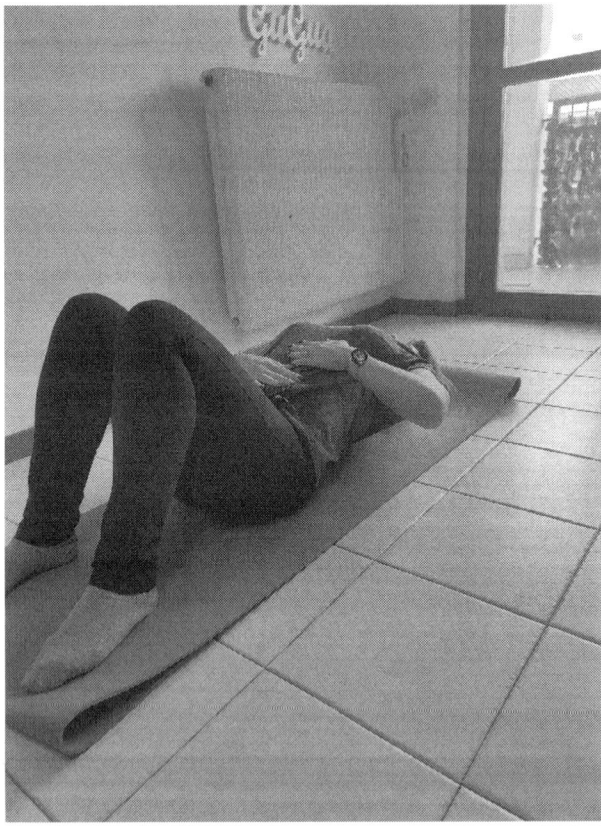

Step 2 - Relax your low back and inhale through your nose (Expand abdominal area and chest gently).

Benefits:

Great exercise to increase the connection with your pelvis and lower back. The aim of the exercise is to help you focus on your breath in a different situation. Inhale while arching and exhale while relaxing. It is suggested to let go of any worries or tensions you might be carrying while performing the exhale for the best results.

How to do it:

- Lie on your back with your legs bent and feet fully on the ground. Place your left hand at the bottom of your chest and right hand on your pelvis, as shown.
- Squeeze your pelvic towards the floor, and exhale fully through your mouth.
- Then, release the tension on your core, and inhale through your nose.
- Keep each position for around 5 seconds. Repeat this movement for the mentioned number of reps.

EAGLE POSE

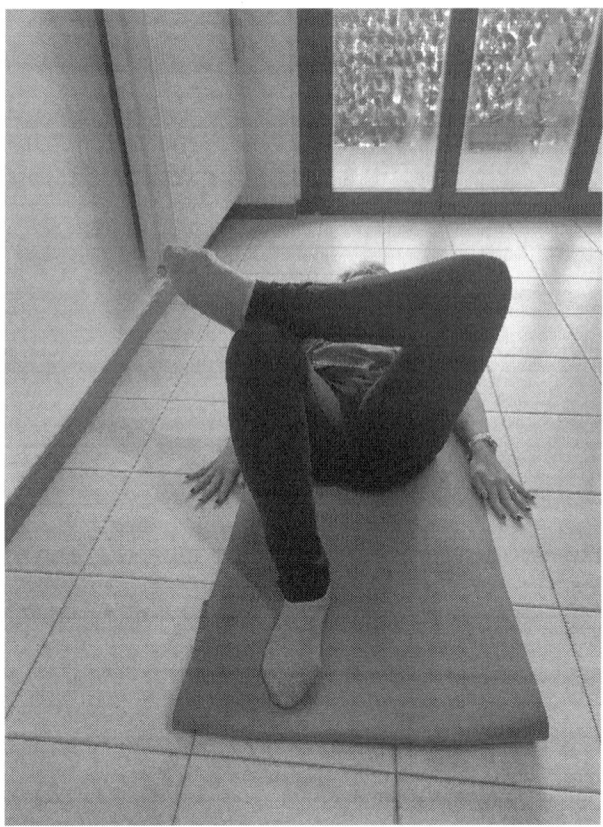

Step 1 - Start with your right foot on the mat, bending your right leg. Place your left foot on your right knee.

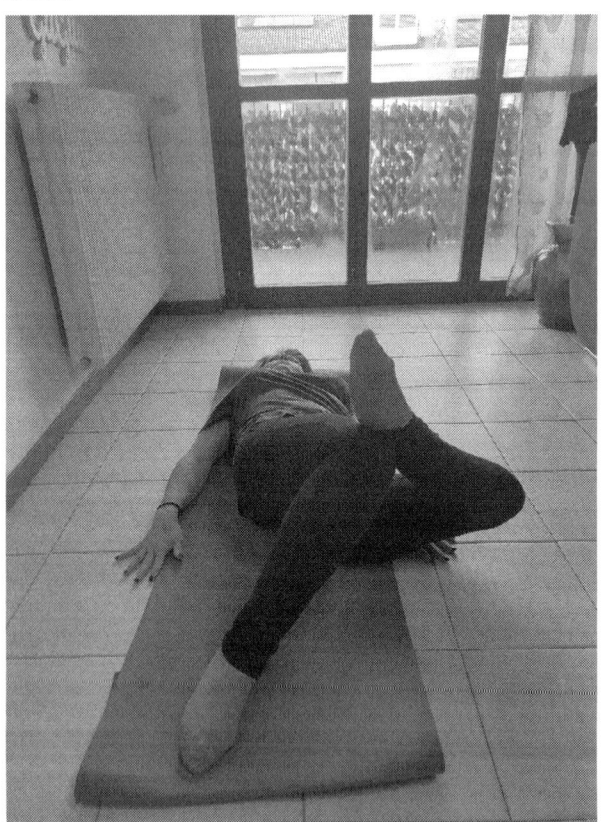

Step 2- Rotate your hips towards the left side. Then repeat it on the other side, switching legs.

Benefits:

Great exercise to increase the mobility of the lower body as well as your back. Relax all your muscles while performing the exercise, especially during the exhale. Breathe out all the tension you are carrying.

How to do it:

- Lie on your back. Bend your right leg with your right foot fully on the ground. Bend your left leg as well, placing the outside part of your left ankle touching your right knee. You should feel a gentle stretch on your left glute. Keep your arms on the floor slightly opened.
- Keep your back on the floor while rotating your hips towards the left side, pushing your left ankle towards the floor to bring your relaxed right leg towards the left, as shown in step 2.
- Remember to focus on breathing. Then come back into the starting position, and repeat on the other side - switch legs as you do that - right foot on your left knee.

MOVING ROCK

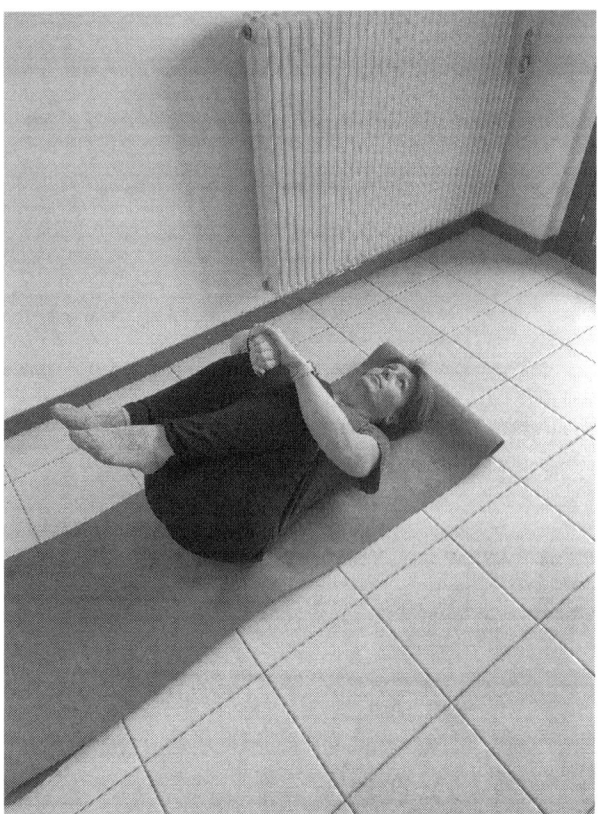

Step 1 - Starting Position, hold your knees.

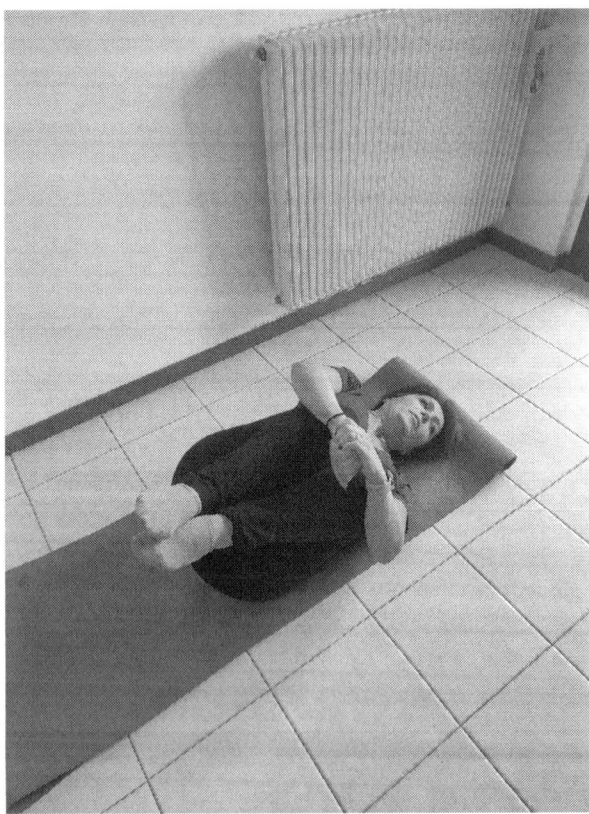

Step 2 - Gently rock to one side. Then, slowly to the other one.

Benefits:

This exercise aims to improve your balance and flexibility. It also requires a bit of core strength. This exercise releases tension and stress in your lower back, making it a great exercise to prevent lower back pain and improve existing discomfort. Focus on surrendering and letting go will help you release stress and tightness.

How to do it:

- Lie on your back and bring your knees to your chest, as shown in the first image.
- Gently rock your body from side to side while maintaining balance. It should feel good and easy. Ensure that your spine remains on the mat throughout.
- Keep alternating the reps from side to side - Move gently and slowly for maximal effectiveness.
- Repeat the exercise for the mentioned time.

NECK AND HIPS

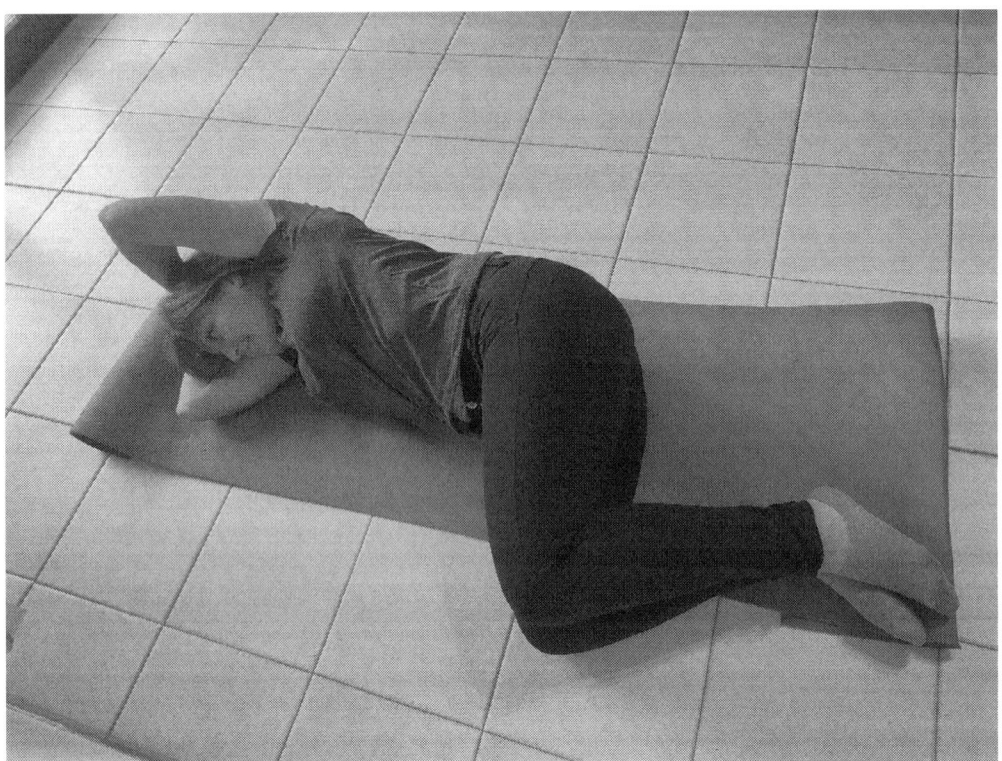

Step 1 - Starting position: Lie on your side with your knees bent. Place your right hand between your head and the mat.

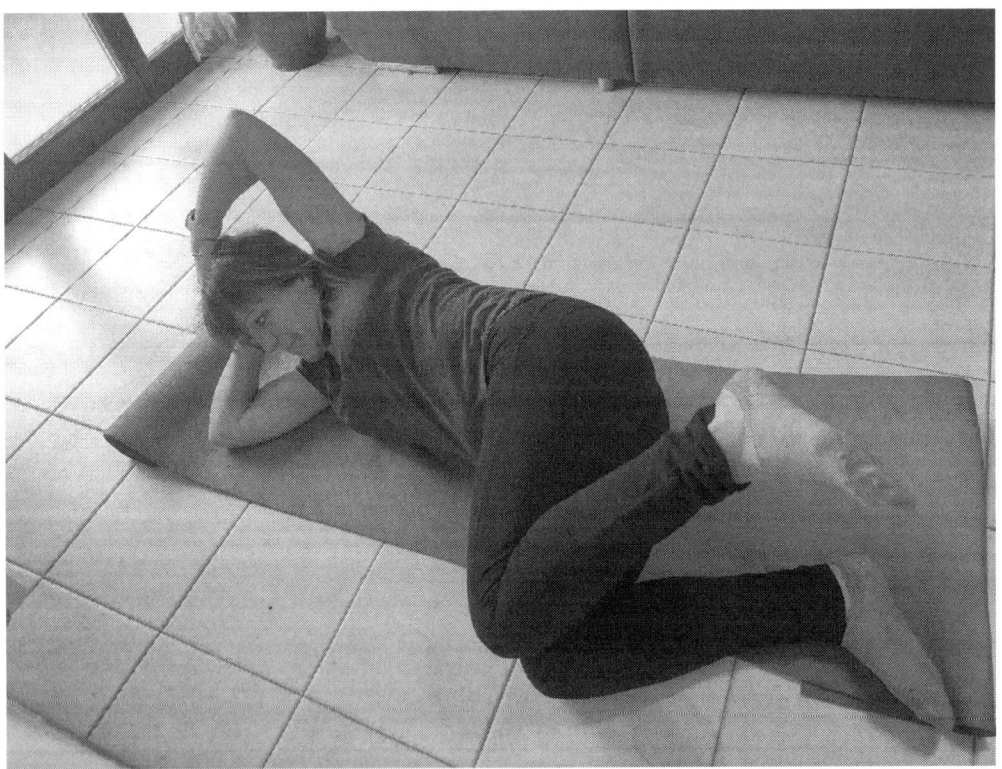

Step 2 - Final position, stretching the right side of your neck lifting it with your left hand. Also, lift your lower left leg keeping your knees touching each other.

Benefits:

This exercise increases strength and flexibility of the neck and the hips. This exercise is very useful for improving coordination and utilizing muscles that are often neglected during everyday life. It enhances stability in your hips and alleviates pain in the neck and low back/hip area.

How to do it:

- Start on your side in a fetal position, lying on your right side with your knees bent around 90 degrees. Place your right hand between your right cheek and the mat, and let your left hand go over your head. Relax and breathe - See Step 1.
- Then, lift your head with your left hand to stretch the right side of the neck. Simultaneously, raise your left ankle as much as possible while keeping your knees together. Hold 2 seconds.
- Lastly, return to the starting position and repeat this movement for the specified number of times.
- At the end, perform the exercise on the other side.

CHEST OPENING

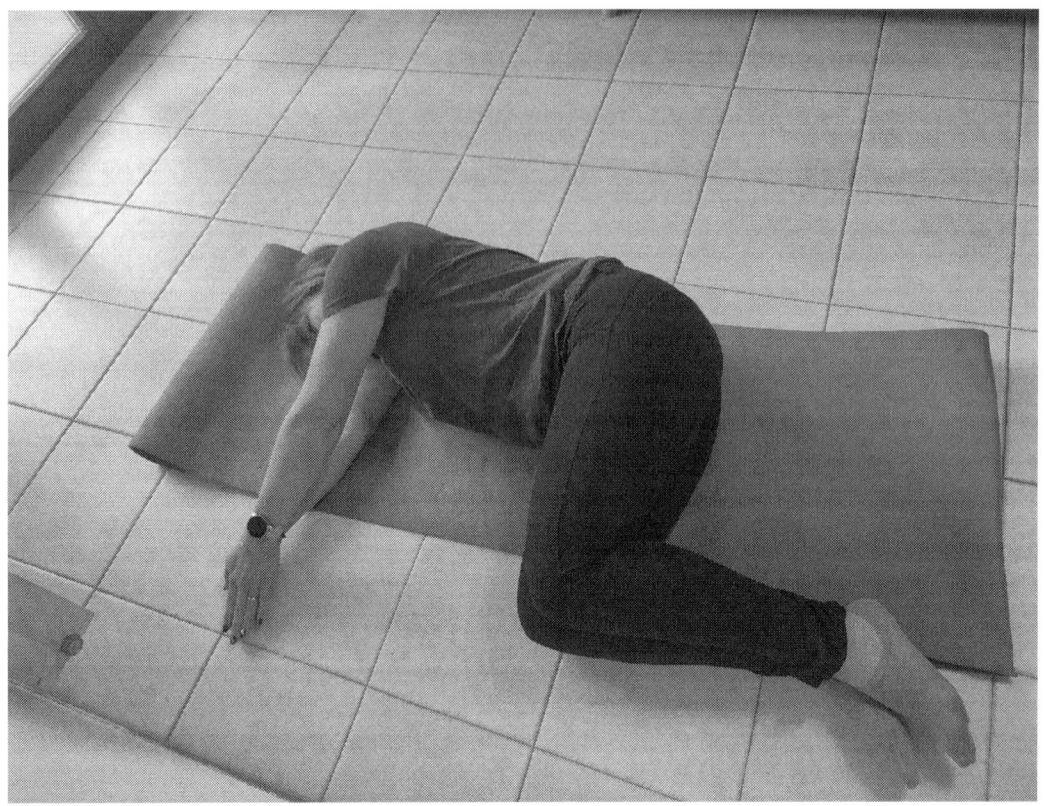

Step 1 - Starting Position, lie on the side with your knees bent and arms in front of you.

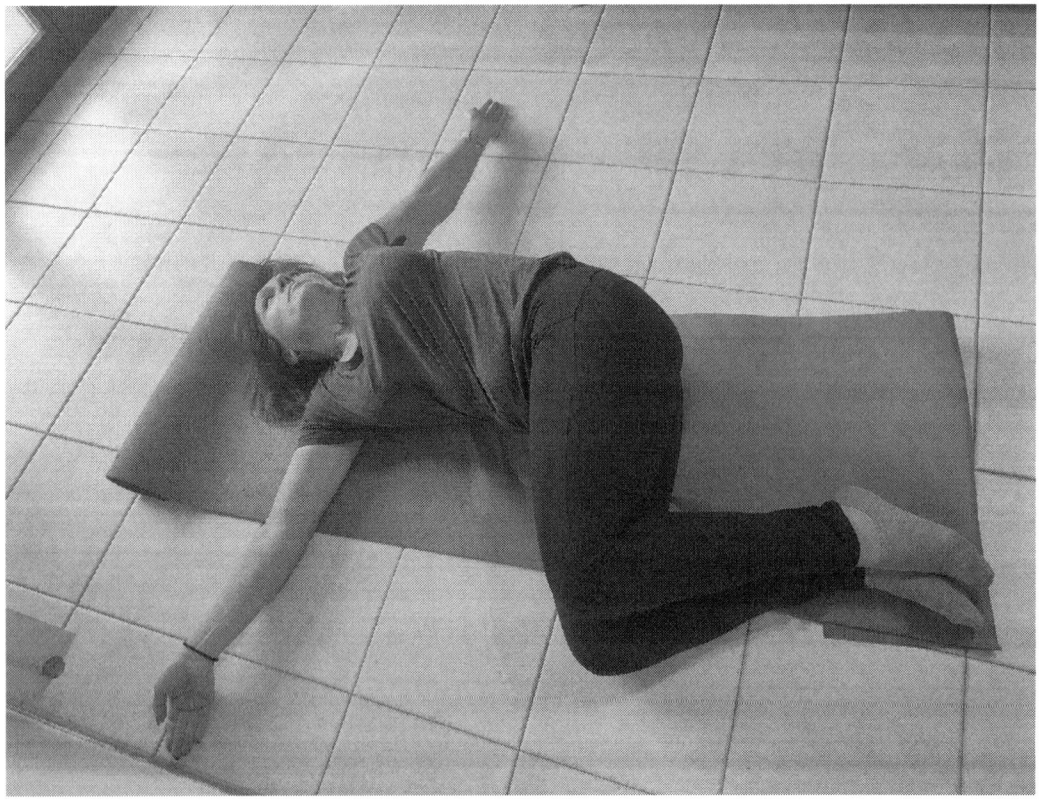

Step 2 - Final position opening up your body towards the left side.

Benefits:

This exercise increases the flexibility of your chest and shoulders while enhancing coordination. Remember to focus on breathing while performing the exercise. It's a great way to release upper body tension. Focus on exhaling to release any tension. It also helps to improve posture and alignment of your body.

How to do it:

- Start by lying on the floor in a fetal position, lying on your right side. Extend your right arm and hand on the floor in front of you, placing your left hand on top of it, as shown in step 1.
- Then, imagine drawing a semicircle with your left hand in the air. Open up your chest while keeping your right hand on the floor, and bring the other hand to the floor on the opposite side. This action will help you 'open up' your chest. Keep the position for the duration of one deep breath.
- Return to the starting position and repeat it for the specified number of times.
- Lastly, repeat the same movement on the other side, lying on the left side.

DESPAIR

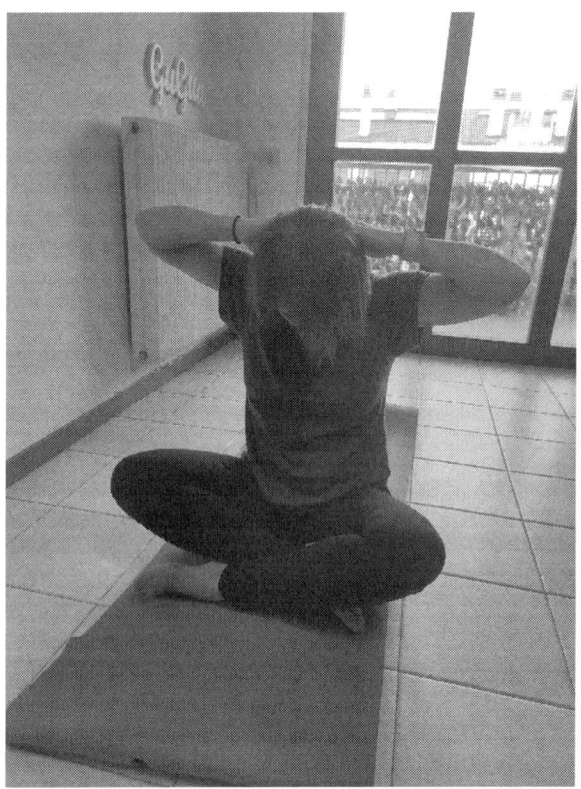

Step 1 - Sit on the mat and drop your chin.

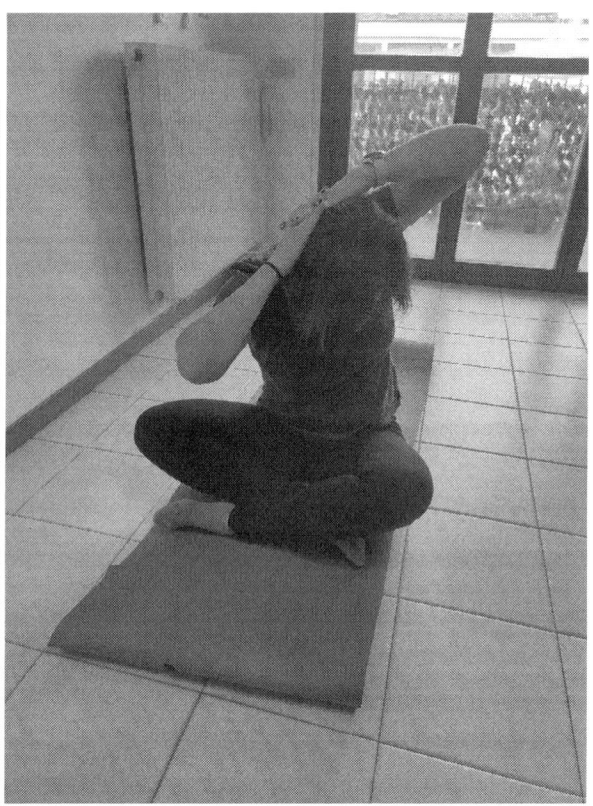

Step 2 - Rotate towards one side and inhale as you do so.

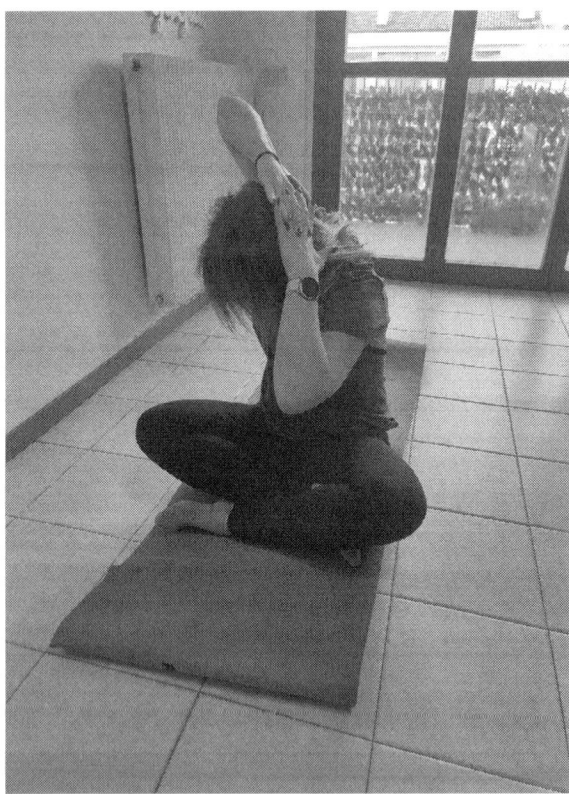

Step 3 - Lastly, rotate towards the other side.

Benefits:

A great exercise to let go of distress and discouragement. These feelings often manifest in the neck and upper body, having a negative impact on the upper body flexibility. If not released promptly, they can cause stress and pain. Also, this position is also beneficial for knee health.

How to do it:

- Firstly, sit on the mat with your legs crossed and your back upright. Place both hands on the back of your head, as shown in the first image.
- Then, gently drop your head until your chin touches the collarbone. Find a comfortable position.
- Slowly, while keeping your hands on the back of your head, turn your face to the left while inhaling. You will feel a stretch on your sides and neck - See step 2.
- Return to the starting position while exhaling.
- Then, repeat it on the other side. This completes one repetition.
- Repeat it for the mentioned number of times.

ROLL IN

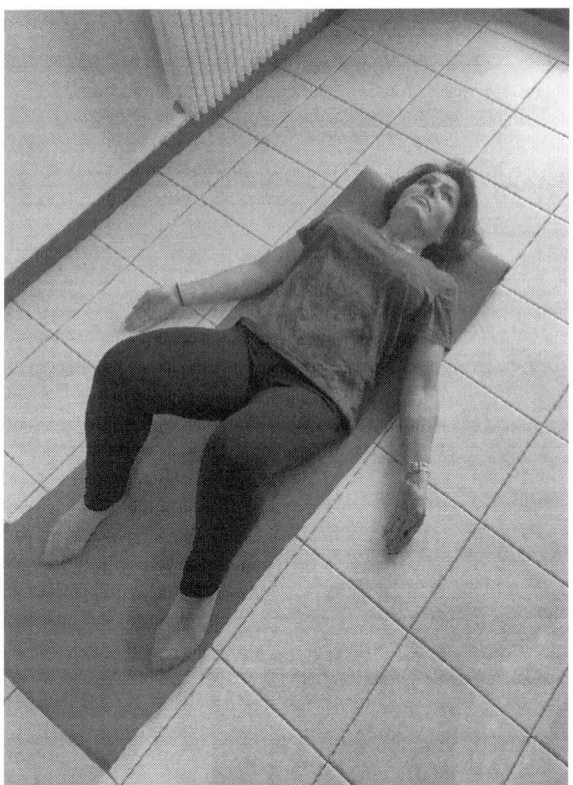

Step 1 - Move your palms facing inward and relax your body. Inhaling gently.

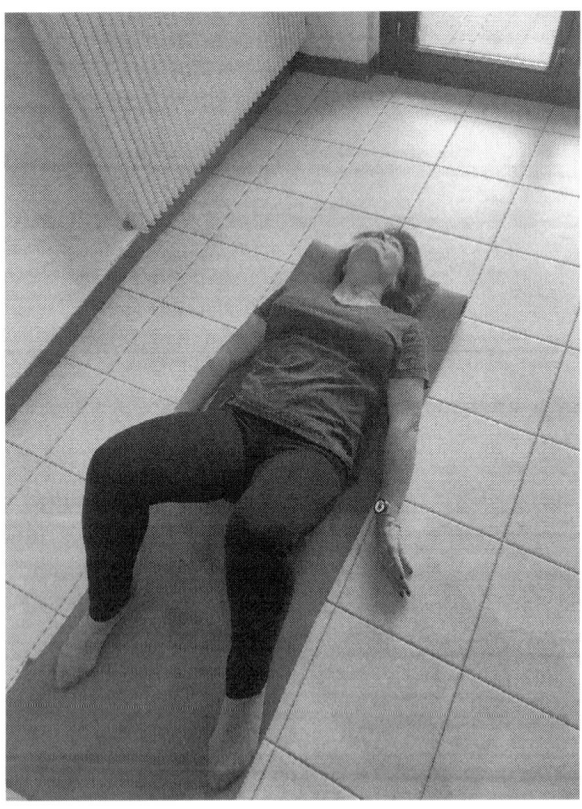

Step 2 - Move your palms outwards, rotate your arms externally and tilt your chin up - Exhale while you perform it.

Benefits:

Rolling in the arms while keeping them on the floor improves shoulder flexibility and mobility. The execution of the exercise might not be easy and natural at first. Once you practice and fully understand the dynamics of the exercise, you'll notice the benefits it brings. Ensure you feel relaxed while doing the exercise. Avoid tensing your body as it could exacerbate tension already present in the body.

How to do it:

- Lie on your back with your legs bent and feet fully on the ground. Keep your arms slightly wider than your hips. Move your palms inward, and inhale through your nose as you do so.
- Then, roll your arms outward while the chin tilts up towards the ceiling during exhalation. Then, return to the starting position.
- Repeat this for the mentioned number of times.

ROLL OUT

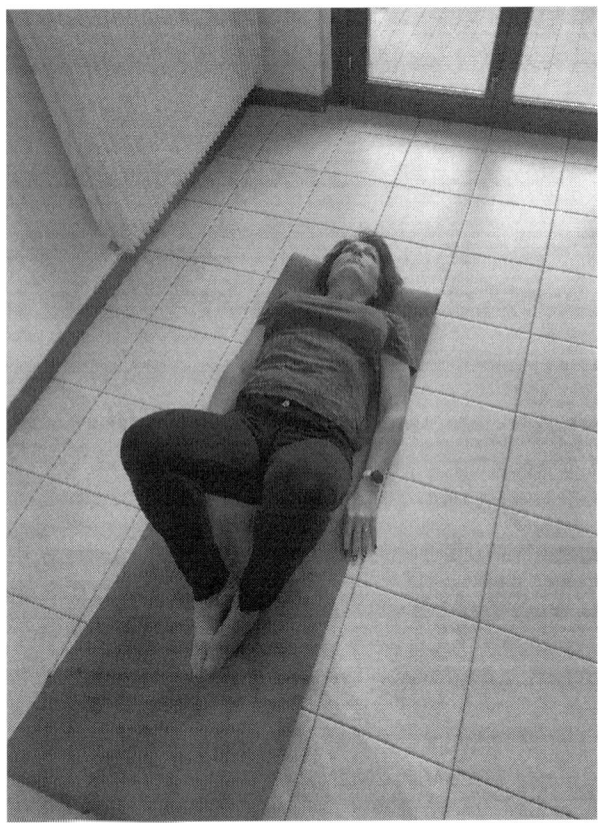

Step 1 - Starting position with legs close to each other.

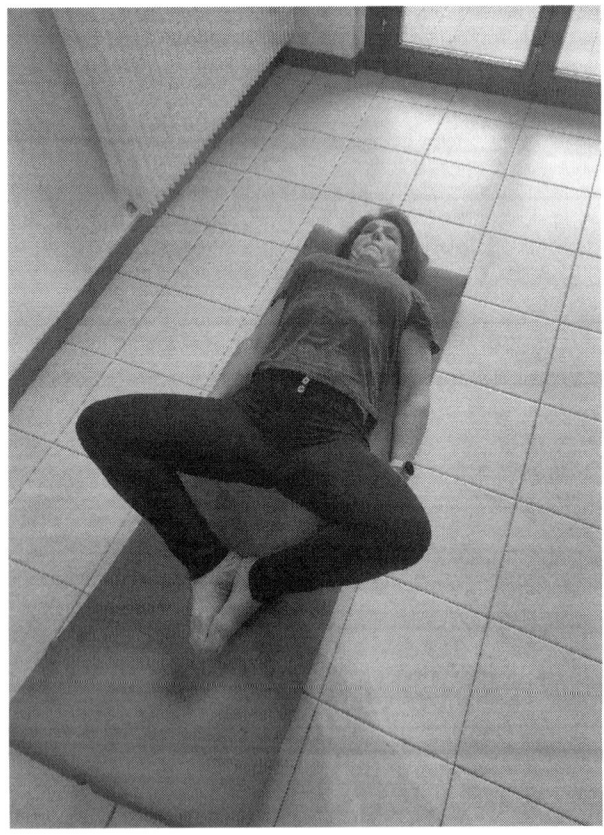

Step 2 - Final position letting your knees drop to the side.

Benefits:

This is a great exercise to increase the flexibility and mobility of the groins and lower back. Stay relaxed and focus on your breathing, you'll perform the movements without contracting your body, which helps maintain a healthy back. It significantly aids posture and enhances the connection with your body.

How to do it:

- Lie on your back with legs bent and feet fully on the ground. Keep your arms on the side of your body.
- Exhale and let your knees drop outward until the soles of your feet face each other.
- Inhale and return to the starting position.
- Repeat this for the mentioned number of times.

SUPERMAN

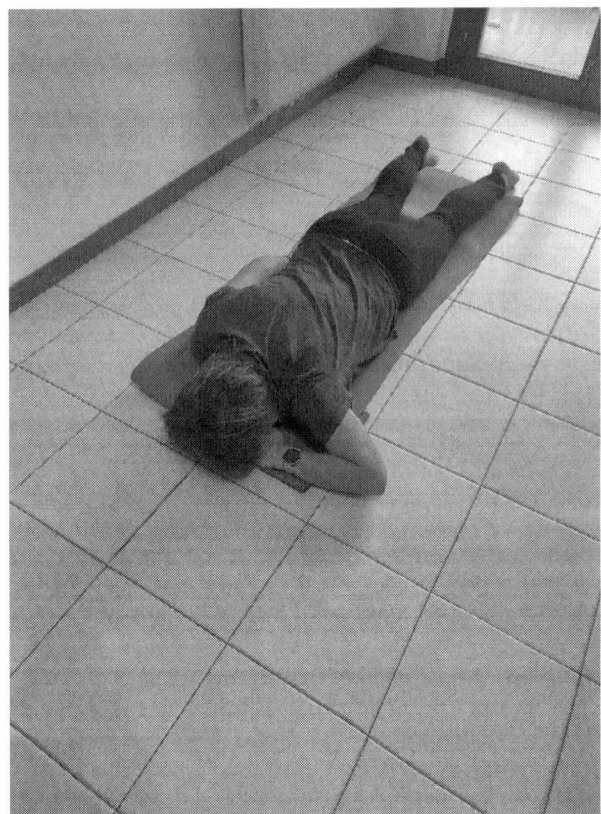

Step 1 - Laying down with your right cheek on the mat, with your face facing the left elbow.

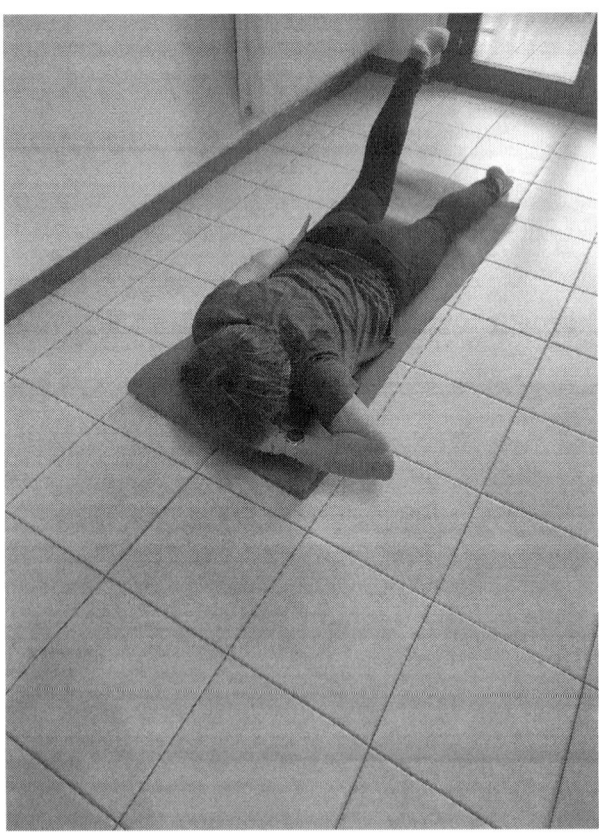

Step 2 - Lift the right leg and left arm. Do it for the mentioned reps, and then do the other side.

Benefits:

This exercise increases the strength of your upper back, glutes, and hamstrings. It enhances the connection with your body by improving coordination. It's a very useful exercise for posture and for strengthening those muscles that are often neglected.

How to do it:

- Relax on your belly, extend your legs, and place your right cheek on the mat with your left hand facing down on the mat. Your left elbow should be relaxed next to your face. Keep your right arm close to your right side - for more assistance, see the first image.
- Inhale and lift your neck and your left arm, allowing your left hand to touch your right cheek. Simultaneously, raise your right leg straight and maintain the position for 3 to 5 seconds.
- Exhale and return to the starting position. Repeat the exercise for the mentioned reps.
- Lastly, repeat it on the other side (lifting your left leg and right arm, facing your right arm with left cheek in contact with the mat/pillow).

SIDE REACH

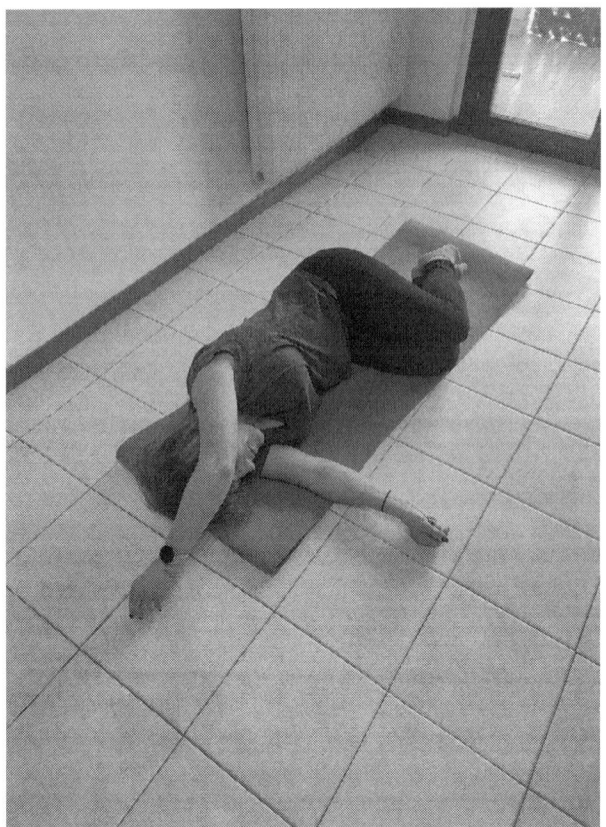

Step 1 - Starting position lying on the side.

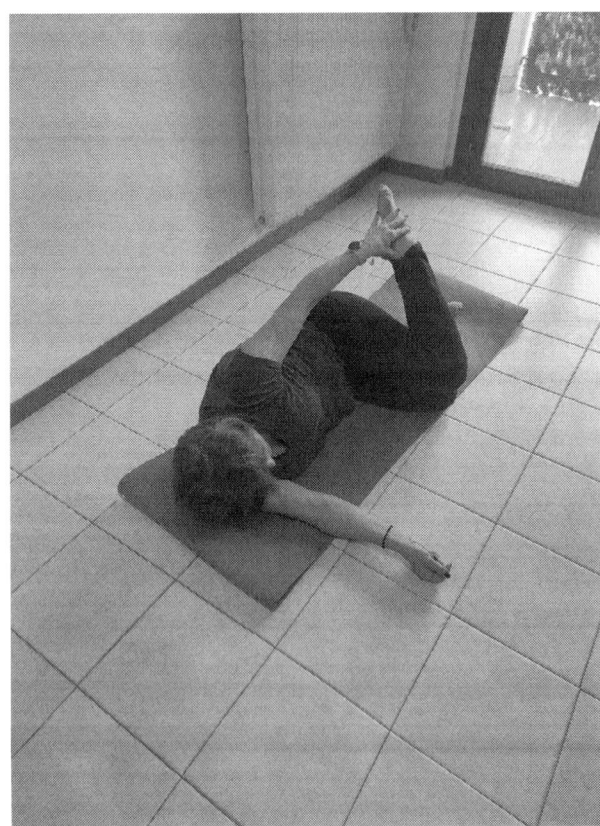

Step 2 - Touch your ankle with the hand that is closer to it.

Benefits:

This is a very fluid exercise that focuses on movement and the fluidity of a motion rarely performed in daily life. This movement doesn't require a particular level of strength or mobility, so it's considered relatively easy. Avoid tensing up while performing the exercise; instead, focus on a controlled and relaxed breathing pattern. For maximal effectiveness perform it slowly and smoothly - exhales always longer than inhales.

How to do it:

- Start on your side in a fetal position, lying on your right side with your knees bent around 90 degrees. Place your right arm in front of you. Extend your left arm over your head, fully stretched - See step 1 for further assistance.
- Lift your head to stretch the right side of your neck while raising your left ankle as much as possible and reach it with your left hand as shown in step 2 - Keep your knees together as you do so.
- Once you touch your ankle with your hand, come back into the starting position and repeat this movement the mentioned times.
- Lastly, perform the exercise on the other side.

SPINAL WAVE

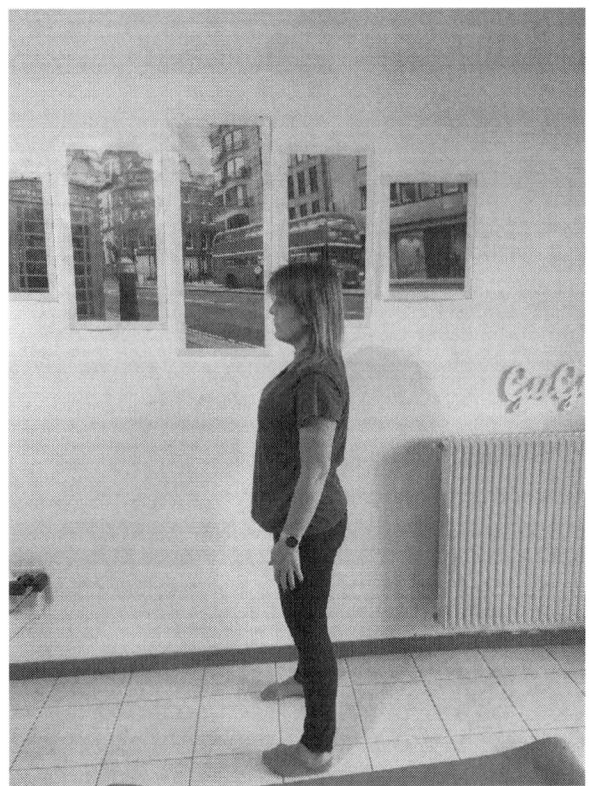

Step 1 - Starting Position standing straight

Step 2 - Move your chest forward gently.

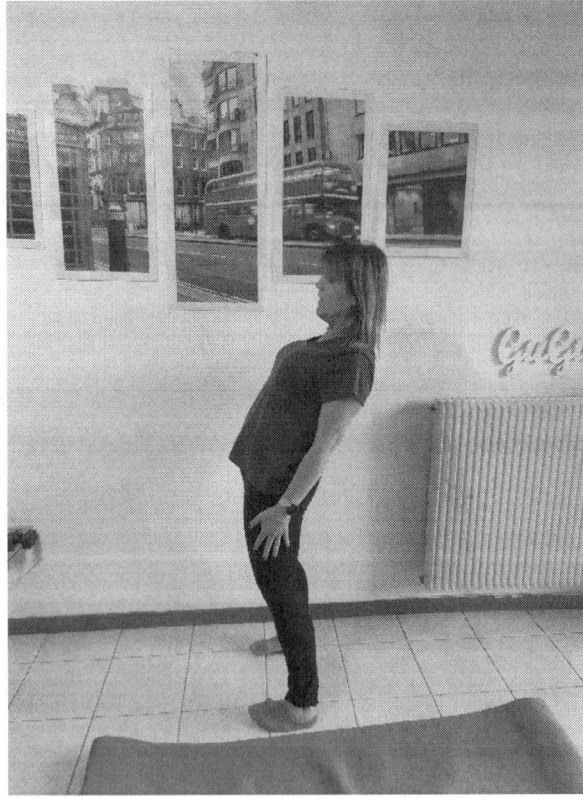

Step 3 - Come back into the starting position and move your pelvis/belly forward. Keep repeating the sequence.

Benefits:

This exercise is great for improving the mobility and flexibility of your spine, preventing pain and stiffness, and releasing tension. With practice, the movement will feel smoother and smoother; it takes practice to master it.
By far one of the best exercises for back health and to improve the connection with your body.

How to do it:

- Start in a standing position with arms on the side of your body and keep your whole body in a straight line.
- Then, move your upper chest forward, Next, come back to the starting position while moving your belly forward, as shown in step 3.
- This is a very fluid movement. Repeat it for the specified duration.

Recommendation:

Still not clear? Let's make it simple: Stand straight while moving your spine as if it were a wave, you'll bring your chest and belly forward alternately.

REACH BACK

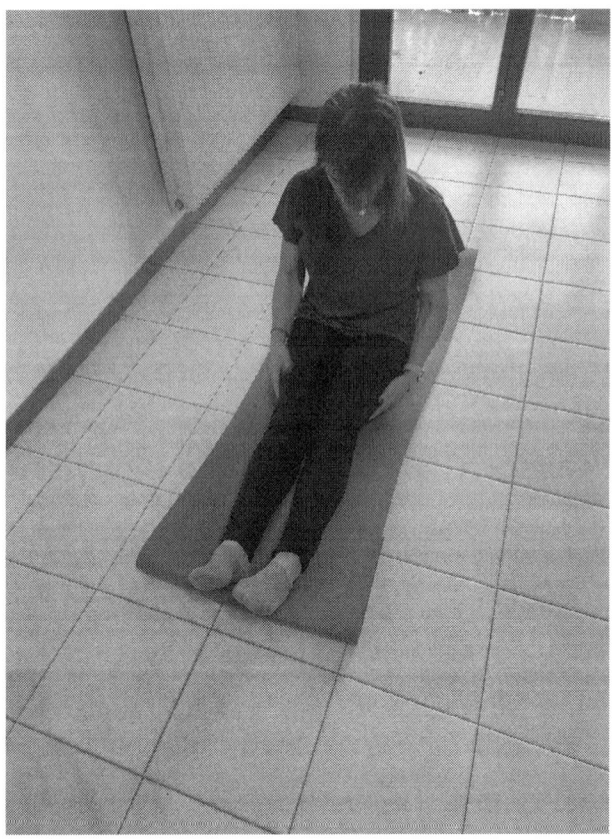

Step 1 - Sit on the mat with your legs straight in front of you and your back straight.

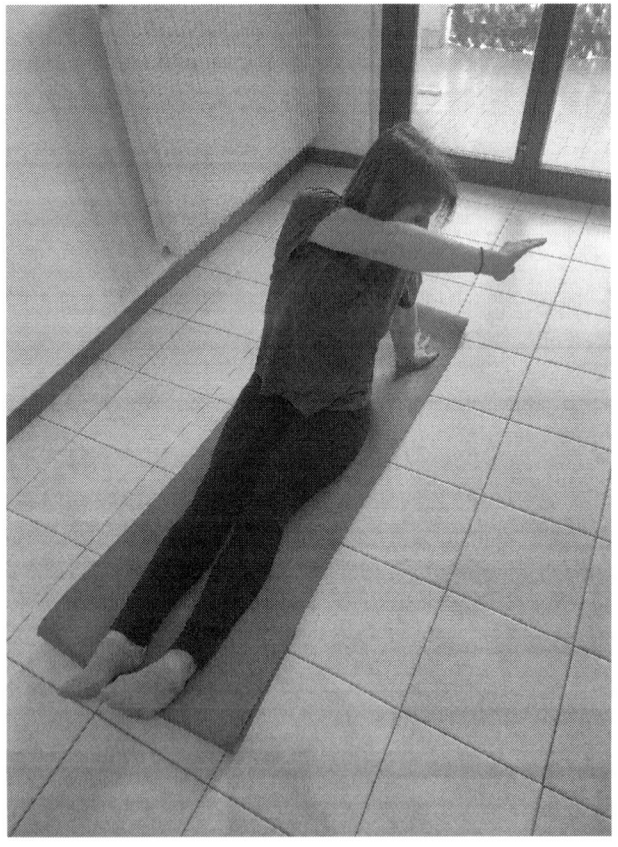

Step 2 - Reach back with your right arm and twist your trunk. Then, repeat on the other side.

Benefits:

This exercise increases the mobility and flexibility of the upper back, shoulders, and lower back. It's important to keep the whole body relaxed and maintain your legs in the same position while twisting your back, head, and arms. Keep one arm on the mat for balance.
Take a deep exhale while maintaining the stretch to fully release tensions and trauma. Focusing on this aspect will significantly increase the amount of stress released.

How to do it:

- Sit on the mat with your legs straight in front of you.
- Twist your back to the left side while keeping the legs in the same position. Place your left hand on the floor and reach backward with your right hand.
- Return to the starting position and repeat on the other side. Keep alternating the reps as mentioned in the 28-day plan.

STANDING REACH

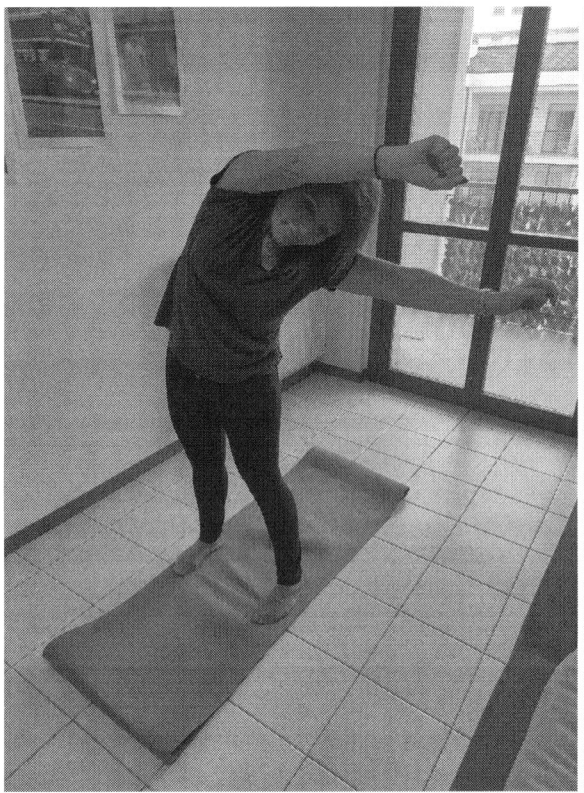

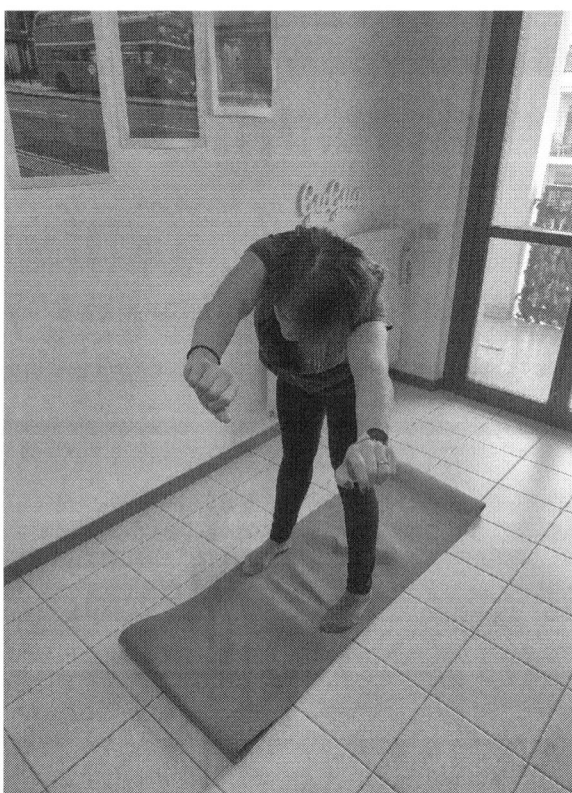

Step 1- Starting leaning towards the left side.

Step 2 - Lean forward, still leaning to the left side.

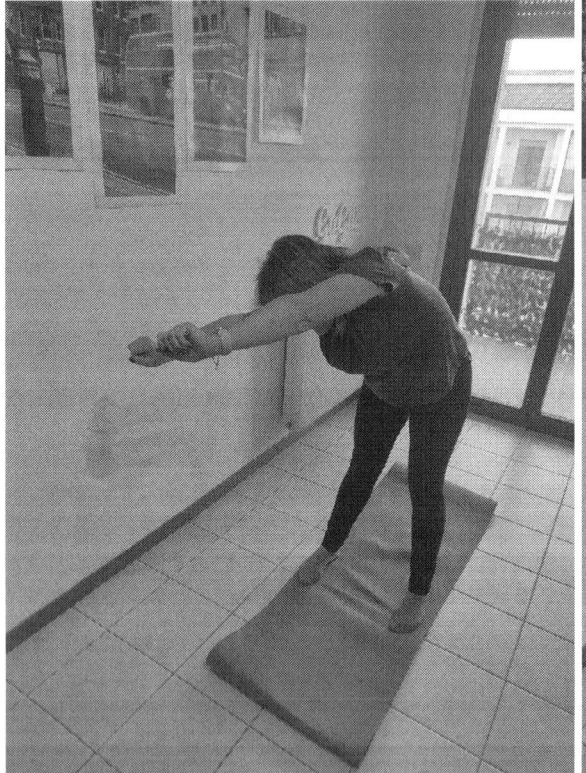

Step 3 - Then, lean towards the right side.

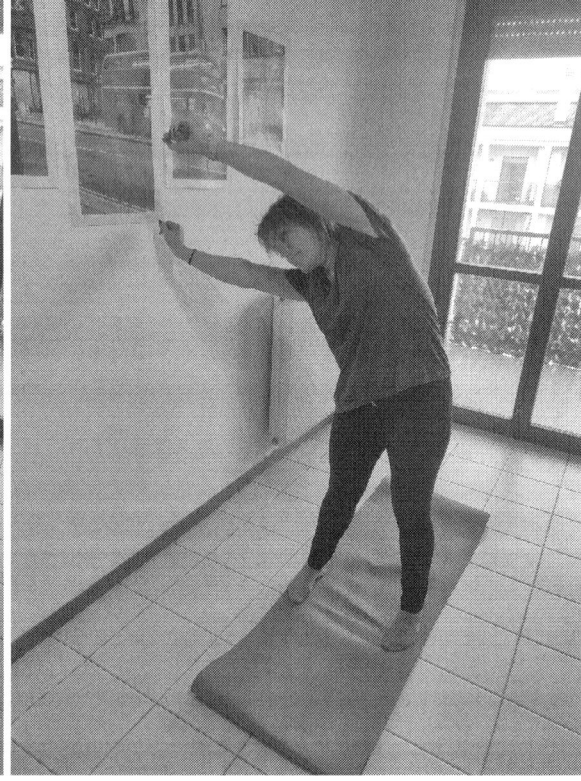

Step 4 - Lastly, lean on the right side. Then repeat the steps from the beginning.

Benefits:

This exercise increases the flexibility and mobility of the upper body. It also enhances the sense of connection and balance you have with your body. Make sure to move slowly and control your breathing as you perform the exercise.
One mistake to absolutely avoid is tensing your neck. Remember to relax the muscles of your neck.

How to do it:

- Stand straight with your hands along your body.
- Extend your arms over head and bend towards the left side while keeping your feet on the floor and your legs straight - see step 1 for further clarification.
- Then, slowly move your hands and torso in front of you to create and draw a semicircle with your hands, as shown in step 2 and 3.
- Continue performing the movement slowly until you reach the right side. Then, slowly perform the movement in the opposite direction. That is one rep.
- Repeat the movement for the mentioned times.

SPIDER CIRCLE

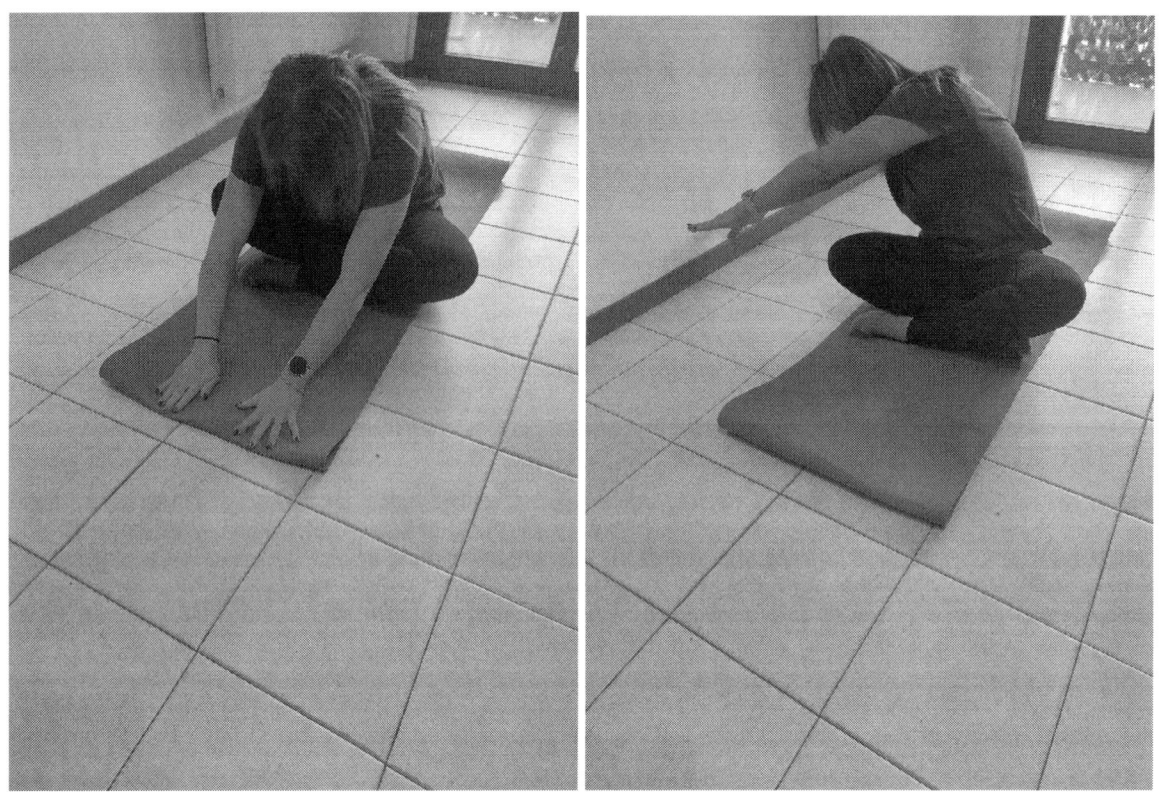

Step 1 - Sit on the mat with crossed legs and reach forward with your hands.

Step 2 - Rotate your arms and trunk to the right side.

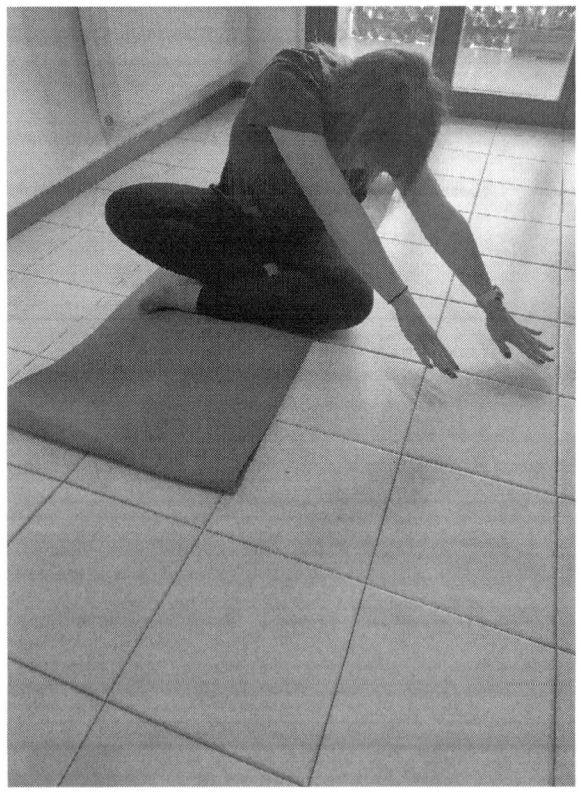

Step 3 - Then, come back to the middle and go to the left side - this is one rep.
Then, go from left to right, and keep doing it for the mentioned reps.

Benefits and Key Points:

This exercise increases the flexibility and mobility of the upper body, releasing tension. It also improves your glutes and lower back flexibility. One mistake to absolutely avoid is tensing your neck. Remember to relax your neck.

Compared to a *Standing Reach* (exercise in the previous page), this exercise does not work on your balance and focuses more on releasing negative feelings. Therefore, it helps more in releasing bad energy and tensions from you, especially traumas and tension, it generates great relief. Let go of worries and focus on the surrender feeling.

How to do it:

- Sit on the mat with your legs crossed while leaning your body forward and reaching with your hands to the floor.
- Then, with a fluid movement, rotate your back first to the right, and then to the left - use your hands to reach as far as possible. That completes one repetition - See image 2 and 3 for better understanding.
- Repeat this for the specified number of times. Lastly, perform it counterclockwise.

STAR GLUTE BRIDGE

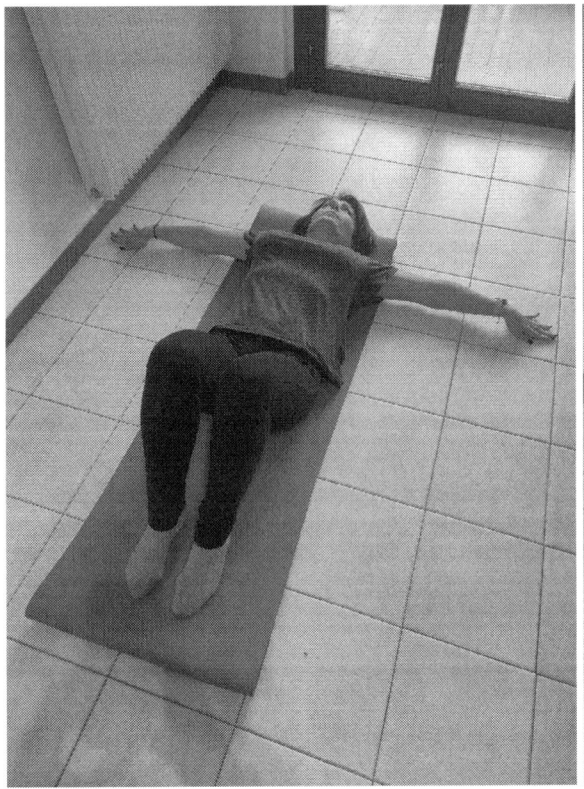

Step 1 - Starting position with feet on the floor and knees bent.

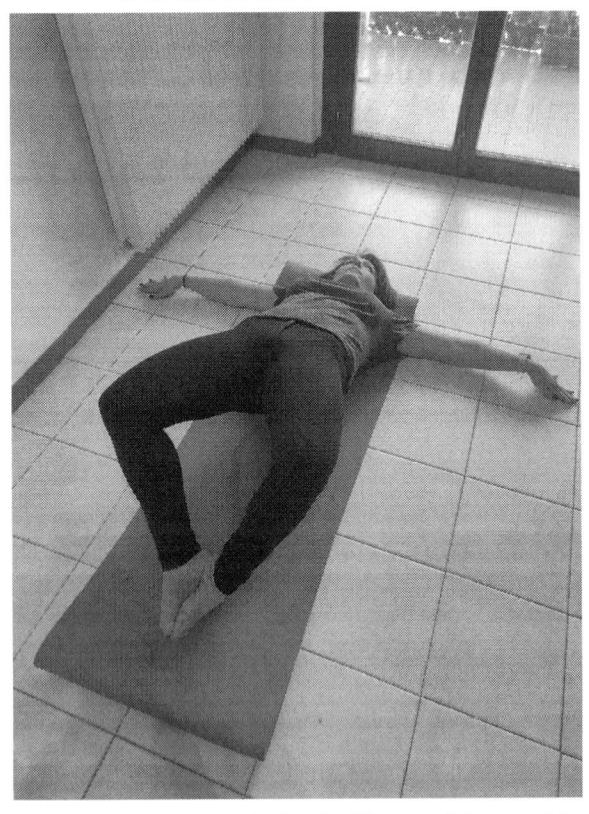

Step 2 - Open up your groin and keep your soles together.

Step 3 - Gently and slowly lift your hips and hold it for 2 seconds. Then, come back into the starting position and repeat.

Benefits:

This exercise increases the strength of the glutes and groins. Engage your core while performing the exercise to ensure you maintain the correct position.
Remember to inhale and exhale deeply to release tension. Relax your upper body and neck.

How to do it:

- Lie on your back with legs bent and feet fully on the ground, close to each other. Fully extend your arms on the side, creating a 90-degree angle.
- Inhale and allow your knees to drop sideways, bringing your soles together. Feel the stretch in your groin as you do so. (you might notice an arch in your lower back- that's fine). Maintain that position for 2 seconds and keep breathing softly.
- Inhale again and lift your hips while keeping your soles together, knees open, and arms in the same position, as shown in step 3.
- Exhale fully and slowly bring your buttocks to the mat, returning your knees to the starting position. Do it very slowly and controlled.
- You have completed your first repetition. Repeat it for the mentioned number of times.

STANDING STRESS RELEASE

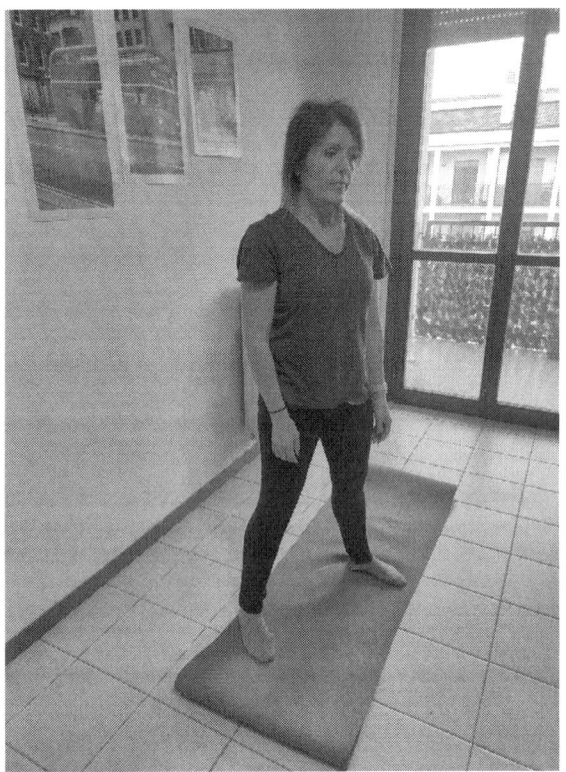

Step 1 - Stand on the mat with legs slightly wider than the shoulder.

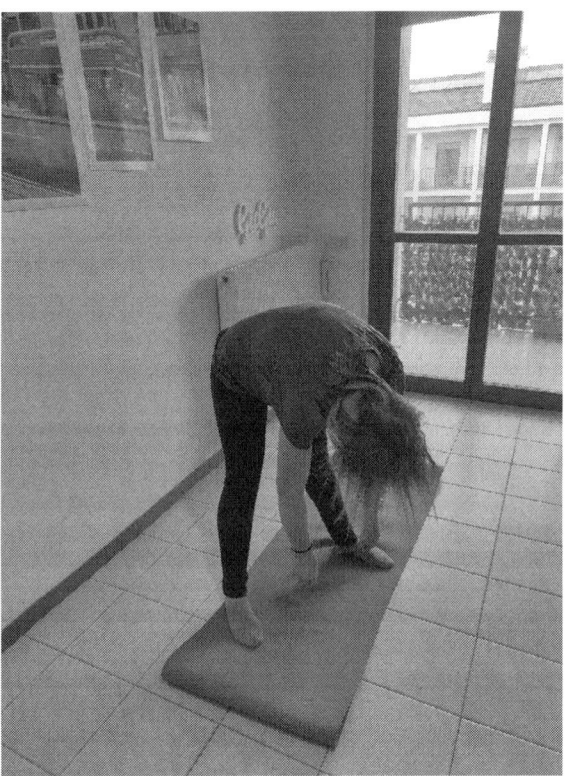

Step 2 - Shake your upper body and release the tension for 5 to 10 seconds

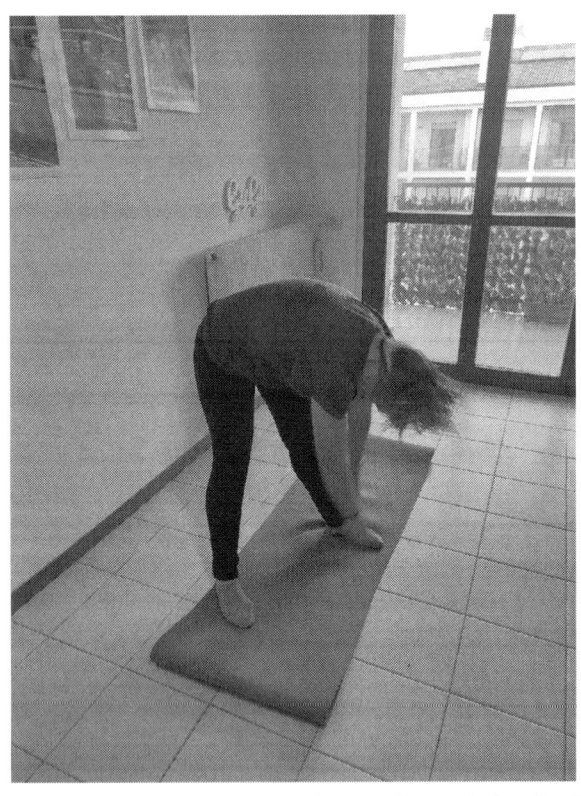

Step 3 - Move side to side gently and slowly. Then, once you shake off your body on both sides, come back into the standing position. Repeat for the mentioned reps.

Benefits:

The key to performing this exercise correctly is letting go. Empty your mind, relax your whole body, especially the upper body.
Imagine shaking off those negative feelings you might be carrying while twisting and turning.

How to do it:

- Start from a standing position with feet slightly wider than shoulder width apart.
- Allow your back and upper body to gently collapse and fall down, as shown in step 2. Let your arms relax and fall naturally. Keep your lower body engaged for balance while relaxing your upper body and head. Fully relax those muscles. Once you find a comfortable position, hold it for 5-10 seconds.
- While maintaining this position, twist and turn towards one side. Hold the position for 2 seconds. Then, slowly rotate towards the other side.
- Come back to the starting position (standing position) and repeat this for the mentioned repetitions.

STANDING SPIDER

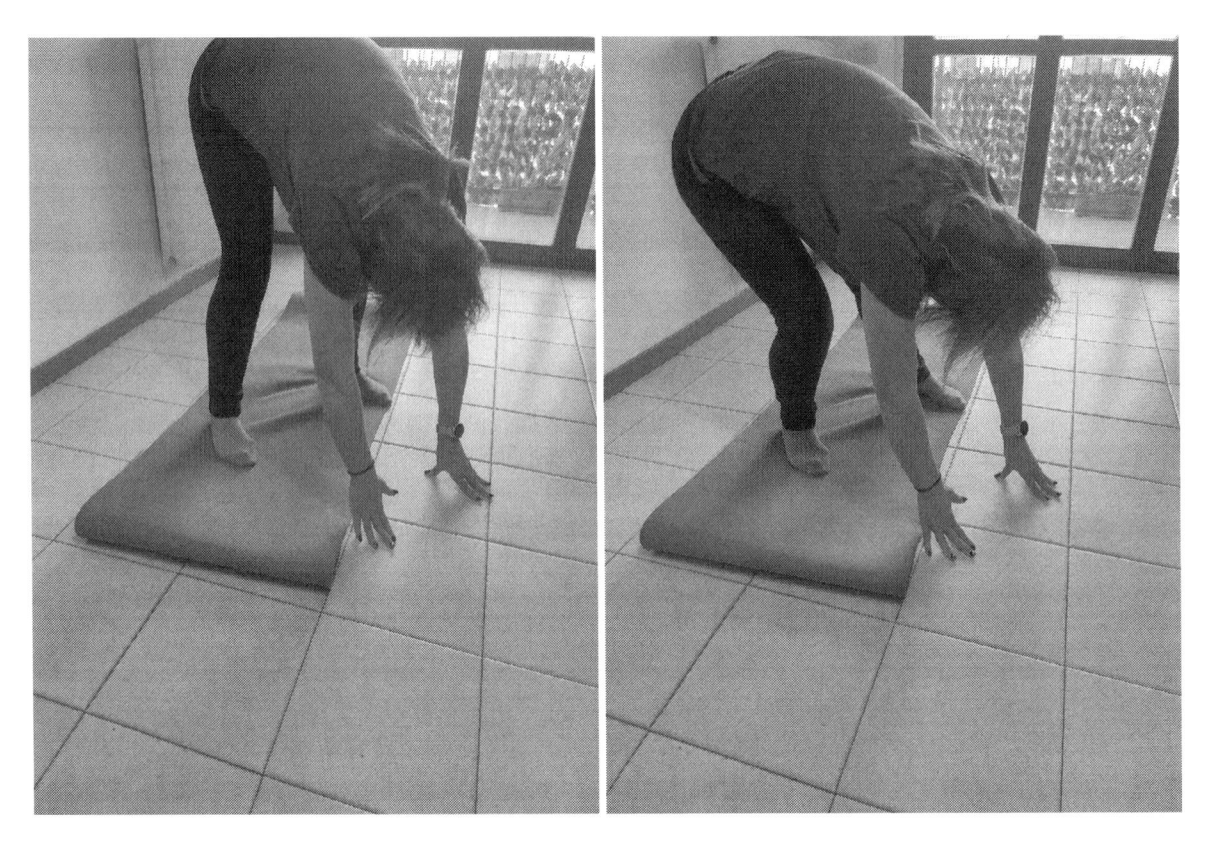

Step 1 - Starting Position, Reaching the floor your hands.

Step 2 - Keep your left leg straight as you with bend your right knee.

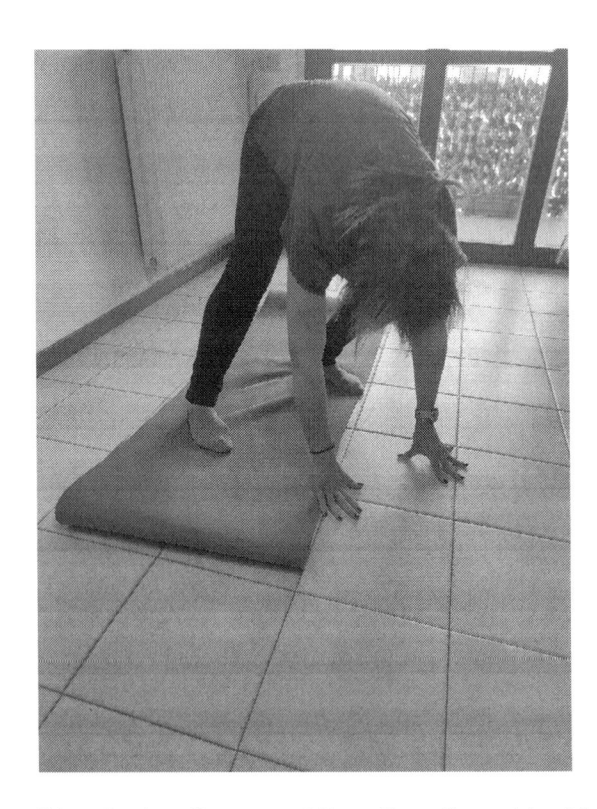

Step 3 - Lastly, repeat it on the other side. Keep alternating the reps.

Benefits:

This exercise is very useful for increasing hamstring flexibility, improving knee health through micro movements in a stretched position that requires balance.

Relax your neck while performing the exercise, and keep your ankles strong with heels on the floor. Overall these exercises release anger and negative emotions that are stored in our posterior chain as well as improving joint strength and resiliency - physical and emotional benefits in one simple exercise!

How to do it:

- Start from a standing position, with feet wider than shoulder width apart. Keep your knees slightly bent while placing both palms on the floor, as shown in the first image.
- Then, perform a very gentle lunge towards one side, bending one knee as well as straightening the other leg - See step 2 and 3 for clarifications.
- Repeat this for the mentioned number of repetitions, alternating the reps.

FULL BODY ROCKING

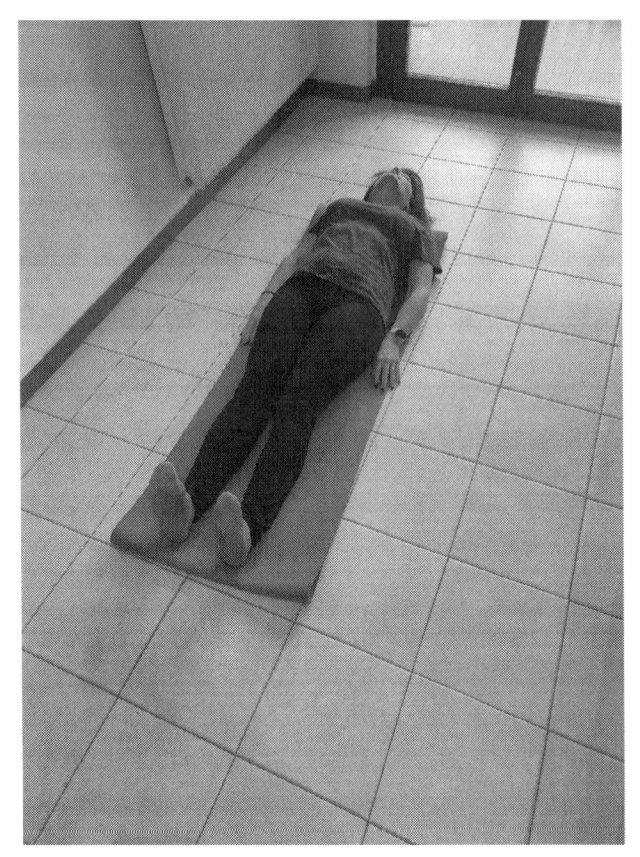

Step 1 - Lift your toes up and inhale gently.

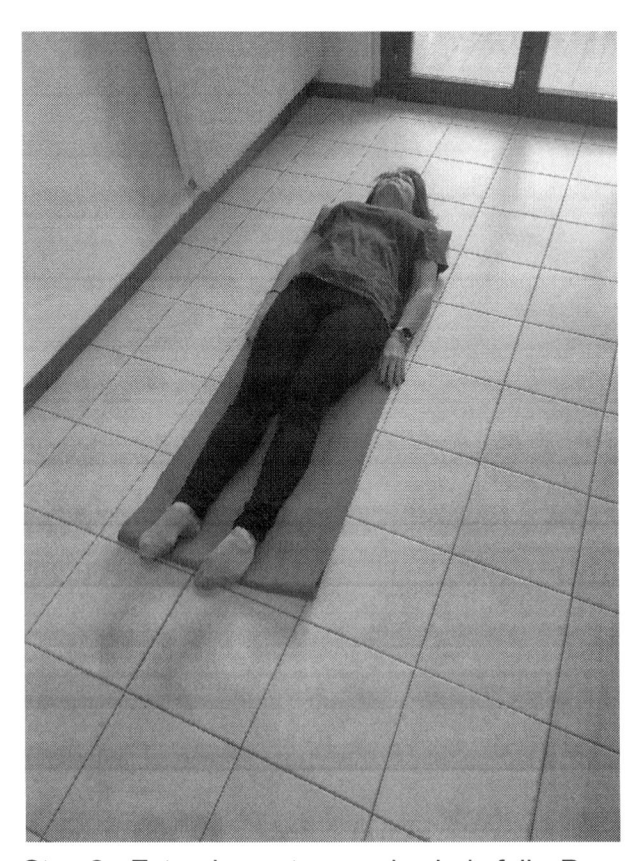

Step 2 - Extend your toes and exhale fully. Repeat the sequence for the mentioned seconds.

Benefits:

This entry-level exercise aims to connect your body from toe to head. If your body is fully linked and connected, you'll be able to feel your whole body getting softer and full of energy as you inhale and relax deeply as you exhale.
The main thing is to pay attention to the foot movement and your breathing. Over time it will be automatic to pay attention to your whole body as you inhale and exhale.

How to do it:

- Lie on your back, legs spread wider than shoulder width apart, and arms next to your body.
- Lift your toes up and inhale through your nose. Hold the inhale for 3 to 5 seconds, feeling the energy going through your body.
- Then, stretch your toes pointing away from you and exhale through your mouth as if you're drinking from a straw. Hold it for 5 to 8 seconds, feeling your body releasing tension on your muscles.
- Repeat for the mentioned seconds.

STRETCH AND COMPRESS

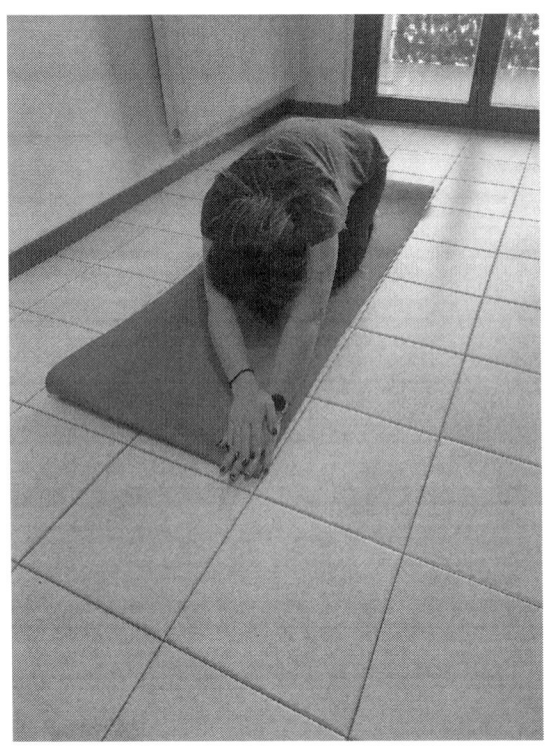

Step 1 - Stretch and extend your arms slightly towards the left side for 10 seconds.

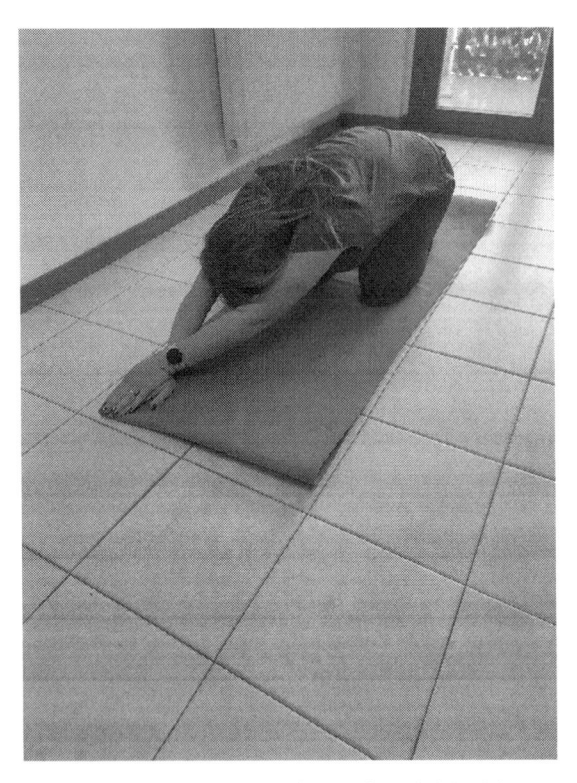

Step 2 - Then, repeat it on the right side.

Benefits:

This is a great exercise to increase mobility and relax your back. Additionally, this position promotes knee and ankle health.
Adopting these primitive and natural positions offers numerous benefits, especially for individuals who spend most of their days seated. It's an excellent exercise to relax, surrender, and feel at one with your body.

How to do it:

- Start by sitting with your shins on the mat, sitting on your ankles and extending your arms out in front of you.
- Then, move slightly to the left side, extending your left arm slightly to the left with your right hand on top of your left wrist. Hold this position for 10 seconds, then repeat the same on the other side.
- Keep alternating the reps as mentioned in the 28-day plan.

ENERGY OPENING

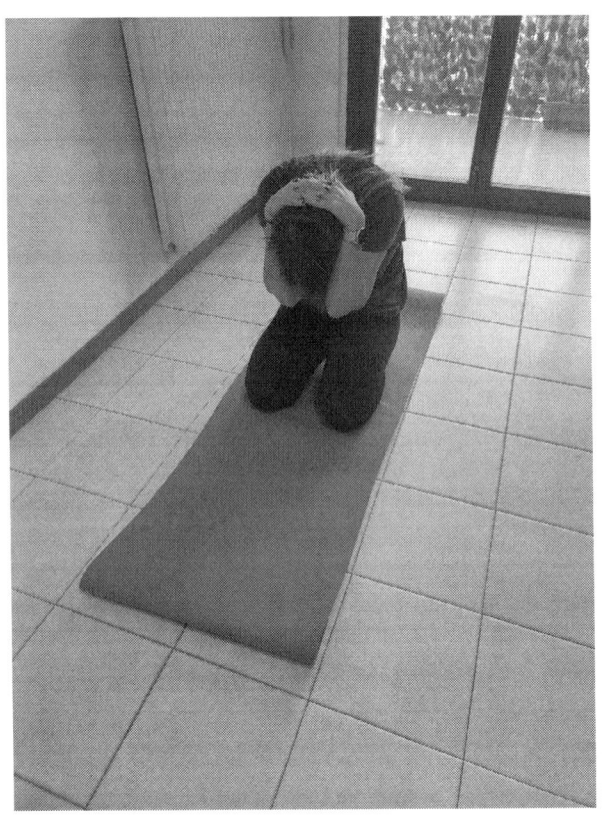

Step 1 - Sitting on your shin, drop your chin towards your collarbone with elbows close together. Exhale releasing all the body tension you feel in your body.

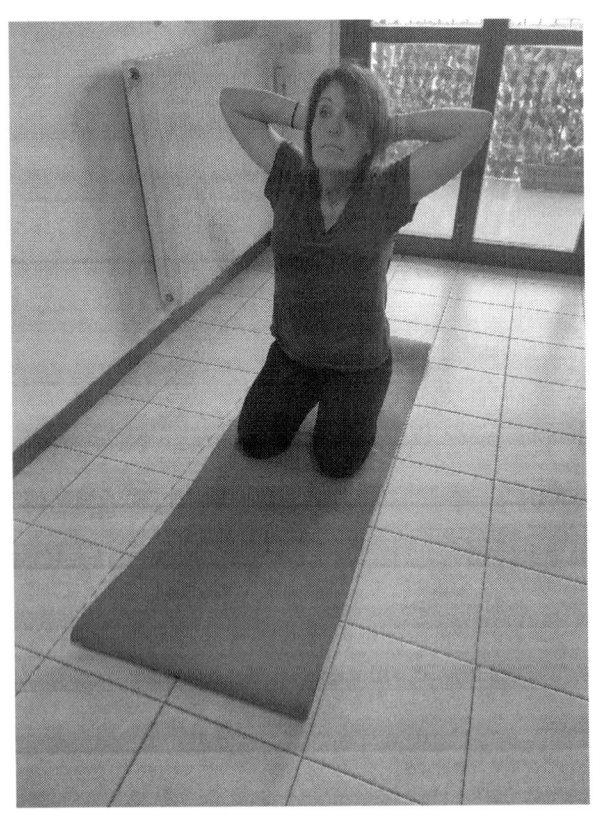

Step 2 - Inhale and open up your chest and arms, feeling your body expand.

Benefits:

This exercise helps to let go of any anxiety and focuses on being present. Release worries and thoughts, and concentrate on the present. This exercise improves your neck and back health, as well as your knee health, by assuming a natural position that is not often utilized due to prolonged sitting during the day.

How to do it:

- Start by sitting on your shins on the mat, maintaining a straight back, and place your hands behind your head, drop your chin towards your collarbone while keeping your elbows closed as in step 1.
- Then, lift your head as you exhale while opening up your elbows and chest. Keep your hands on the back of your head.
- Exhale as you come back into the initial step.
- Repeat this for the mentioned number of repetitions.

KNEE HOLD

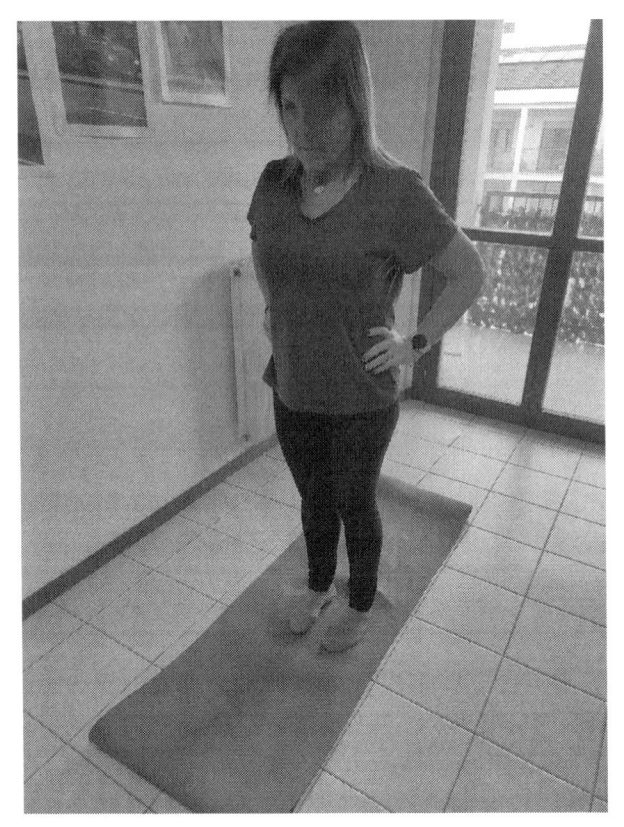

Step 1 - Stand on the mat.

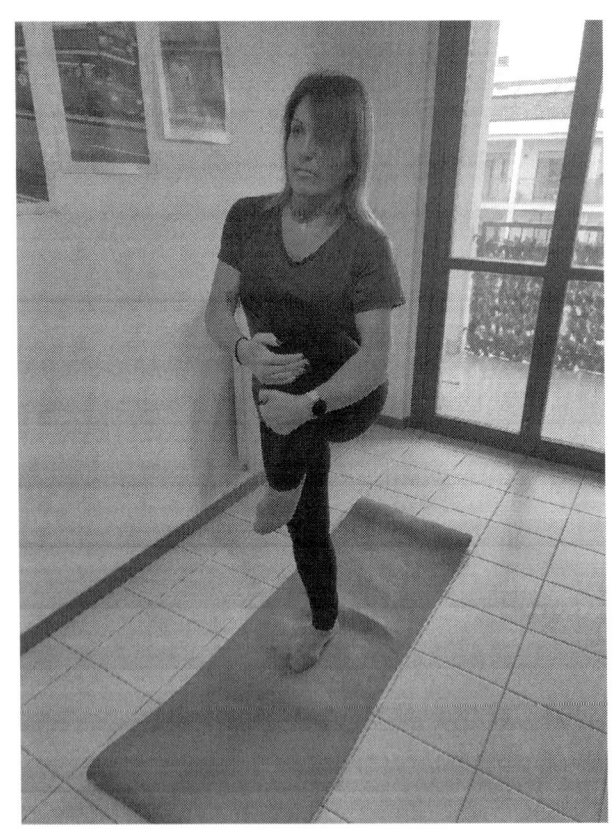

Step 2 - Hold your knee up for 10 seconds - Keep breathing as you do so. Then, repeat with the other leg.

Benefits:

This exercise improves coordination and balance while increasing mobility in the lower body. It's a great exercise to find your center and feel in charge of your body and emotions. It feels good 'hugging' your leg and helps increase positive emotions over negative ones. Additionally, it improves the strength of your arms and upper body.

How to do it:

- Start by standing on the mat.
- Then, bring one knee close to your chest with both hands, keeping only one foot on the floor - if you lack balance try focusing on observing a specific point on the floor a few feet away from you. "Fixing" your eyes on something usually helps you feel more balanced.
- Focus on deep and controlled breathing, inhaling through your nose and exhaling through your mouth
- Maintain the position for 10 seconds - Keep breathing gently as you do so.
- Repeat this for the mentioned number of repetitions, alternating the side.

NECK RELEASE

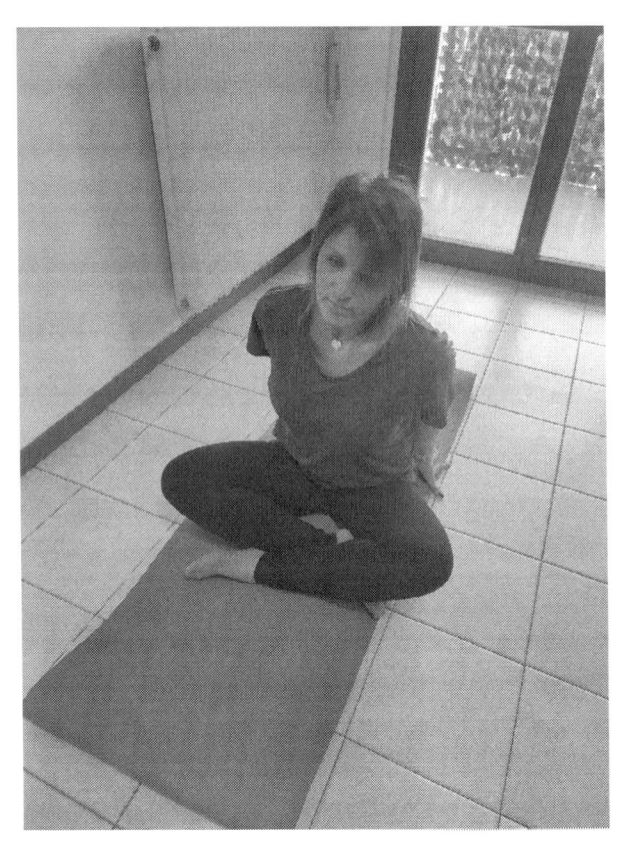

Step 1 - Sit on the mat with crossed legs and a straight back.

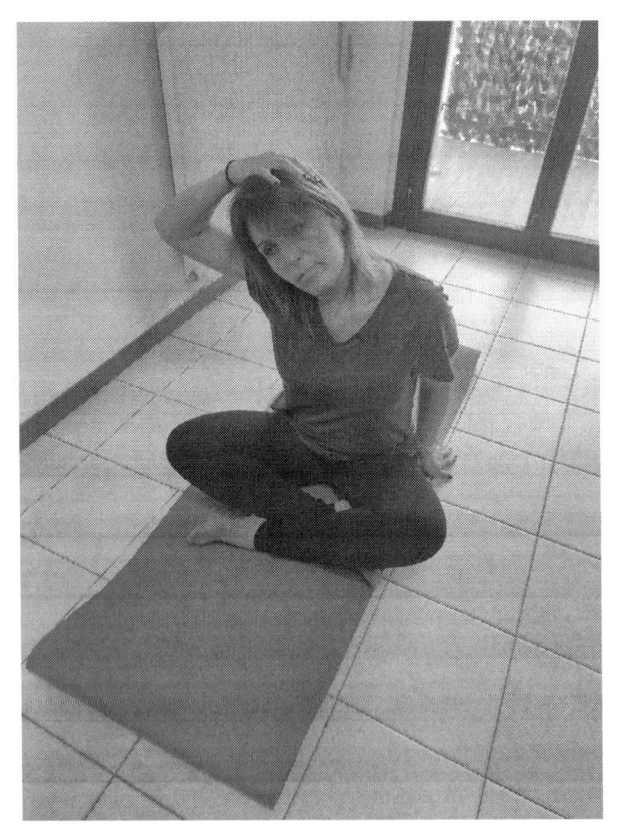

Step 2 - Stretch your neck for 5 seconds, then repeat it on the other side. Perform it for the mentioned reps.

Benefits:

Releasing your neck helps you release stress, gives you energy, and makes you feel less tense.
This exercise mainly aims to release neck tension. It stretches your neck, improving flexibility, posture, and alignment, especially for individuals who use laptops or smartphones frequently and tend to keep their necks in a non-straight position.

How to do it:

- Sit on the mat with your legs crossed.
- Then, reach with your right hand over your head and pull the left side of your head towards your right shoulder. This action will create a stretch in the left side of your neck. Hold it for 5 seconds - Keep breathing gently and softly.
- Lastly, repeat it on the other side, alternating the reps from left to right side.

OPEN LIFE

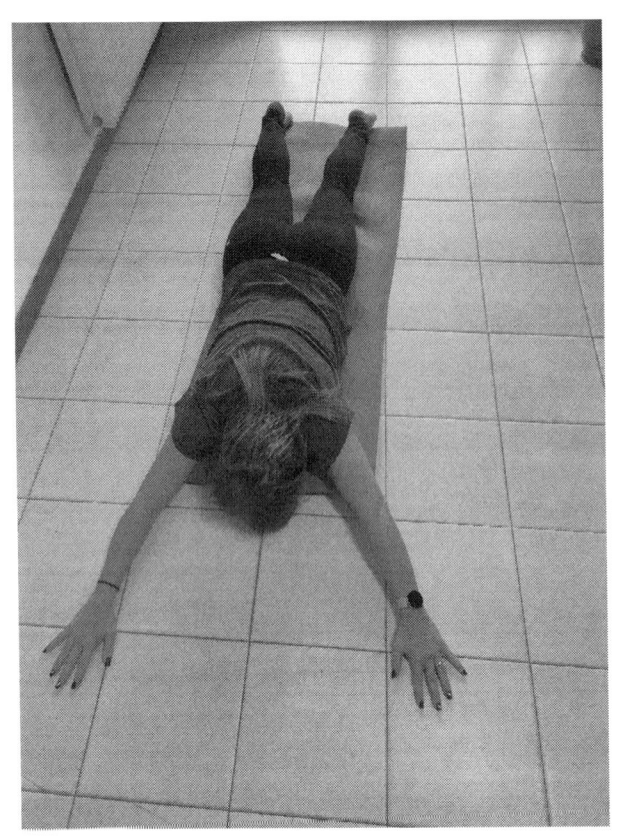

Step 1 - Starting position, extend your arms and legs and relax.

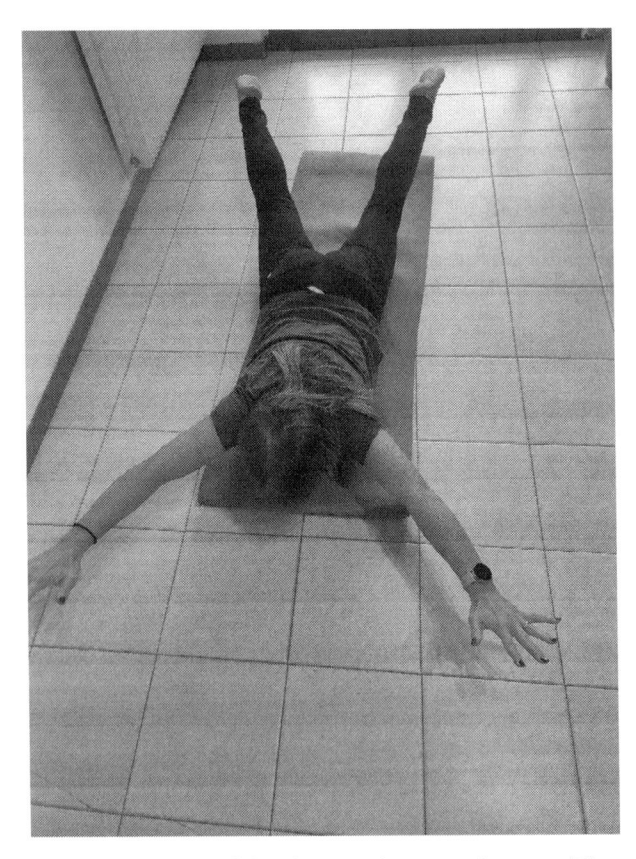

Step 2 - Then, lift both your legs and arms. Then, come back into the starting position.

Benefits:

This exercise helps increase energy and happiness. It's a great exercise that makes you feel in charge and in control of your body, while also increasing the strength of both your upper and lower body. As a grounding exercise, it helps you feel more connected with your heart. Additionally, it improves posture and body alignment.

How to do it:

- Lie on your belly on the mat with legs extended and relaxed, ankles relaxed, and arms stretched in front of you. Relax all muscles from neck to ankles.
- Inhale and lift your arms and legs as much as possible while keeping your pelvis and core on the mat - hold it for 2 seconds.
- Return to the starting position, and perform the exercise for the specified number of reps.

JUMPING JACKS

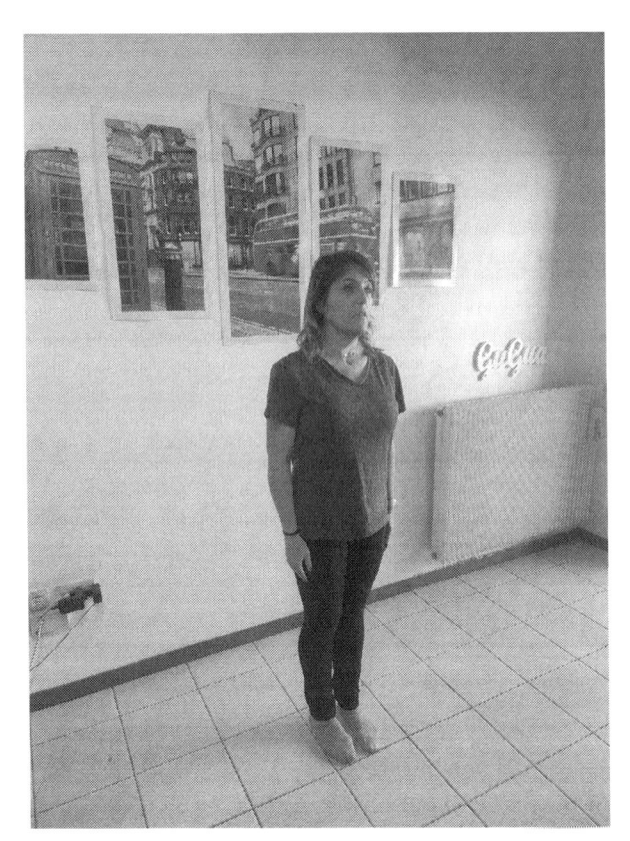

Step 1 - Start standing with feet close to each other and arms next to the body.

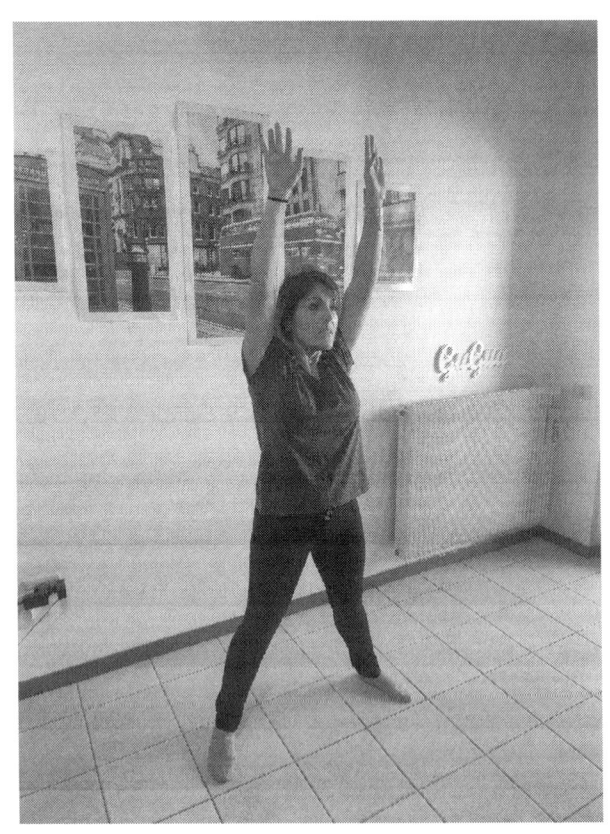

Step 2 - Jump and open your legs while lifting your arms straight above your head. Then, come back into the starting position and repeat the movement for the mentioned seconds.

Benefits:

Jumping Jacks are a full-body exercise that can help you burn a lot of calories in a short time, making them great for weight loss. It's important to focus on breathing while performing the exercise. When exhaling, you'll release any negative emotions you might be carrying.

How to do it:
- Start by standing on the mat with your legs close together and your arms resting alongside your body.
- Next, make a small jump while simultaneously opening your legs wide and your arms over your head.
- Then, perform another small jump to return to the starting position. This sequence completes one repetition.
- Repeat this exercise for the mentioned period of time.

BURPEES

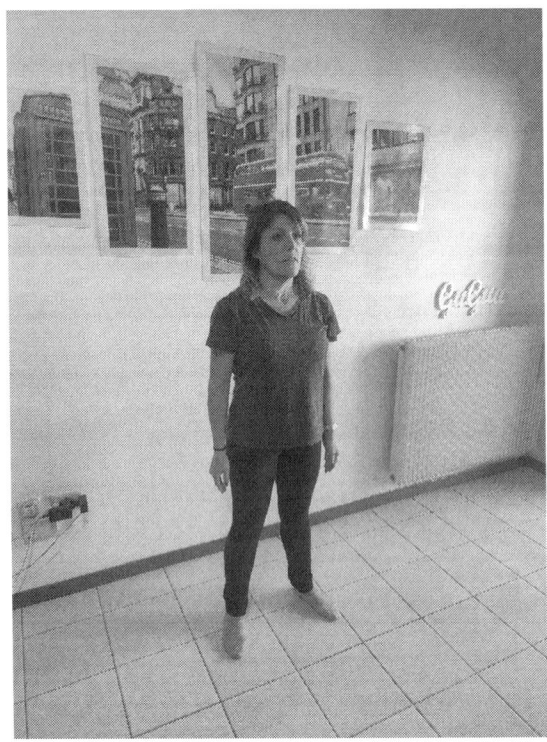

Step 1 - Start standing with feet shoulder width apart and arms next to the body.

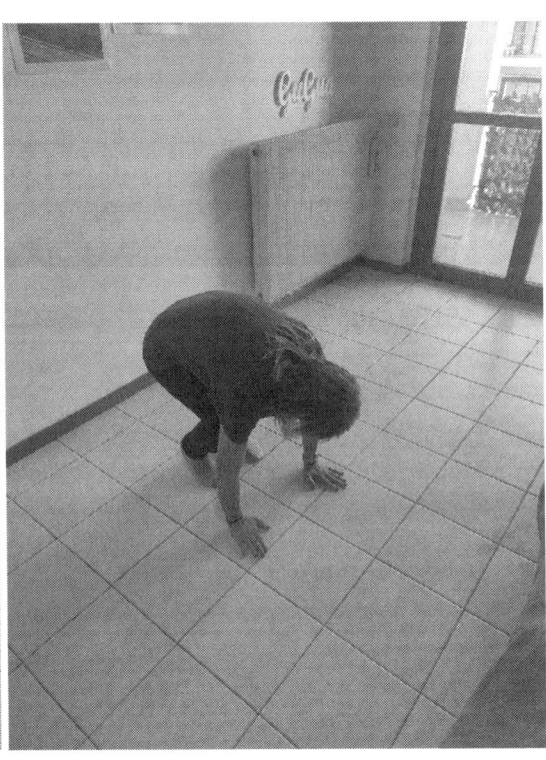

Step 2 - Keep your feet on the floor, bring your hands on the floor.
Bend your knees, preparing yourself to move into a push-up position.

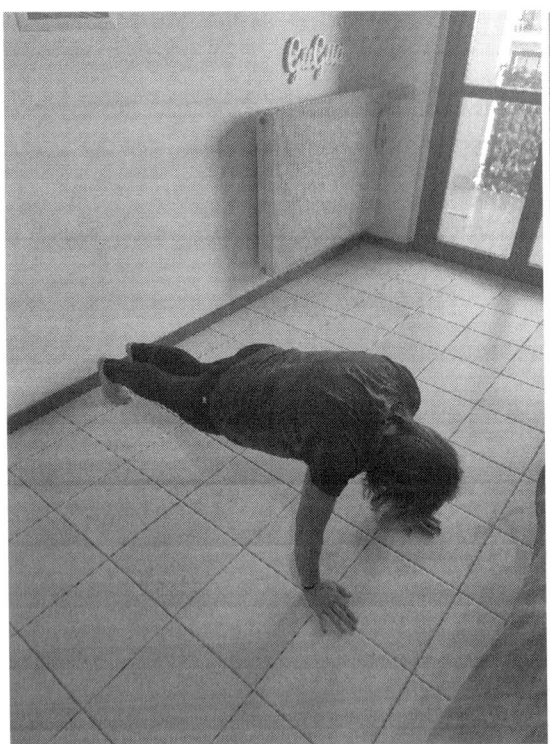

Step 3 - Straighten your legs back, either Jump or one foot at a time.

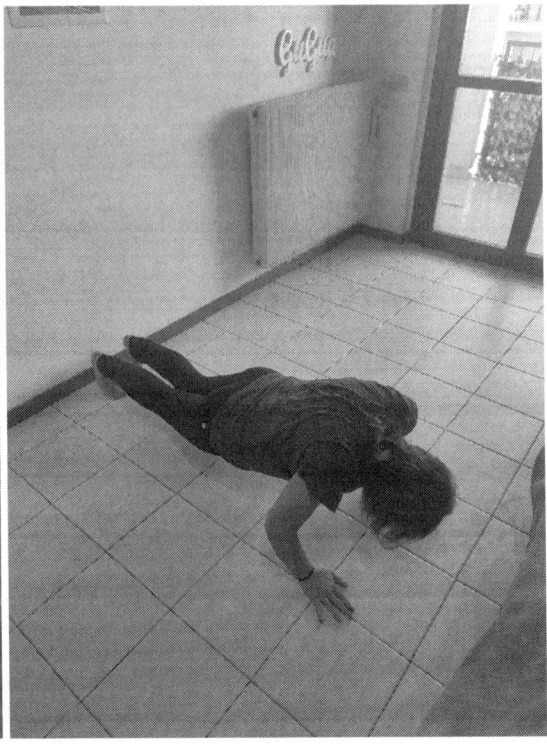

Step 4 - Perform a push-up and repeat it (see explanation for easier version).

Benefits:

Burpees engage every part of your body, resulting in a high calorie burn and rapid weight loss. It is crucial to keep your attention on your breath throughout this exercise. When returning to the starting position after completing a repetition, exhaling helps release any negative and repress emotion. It's critical to exhale right away and completely to get rid of tension.

How to do it:
- Begin by standing on the mat with your legs shoulder-width apart and your arms relaxed by your sides Step 1.
- Next, move your hands on the floor -bend your knees as you do so - Step 2.
- Lastly, get in a push-up position - Step 3. Either jumping back with your legs or bringing your legs back one at a time.
- Perform a push-up as shown in Step 4 or simply get your chest and core on the floor, and then come back up in a push-up position.
- Following that, stand up again, you just completed one repetition.
- Repeat this exercise for the mentioned period of time.

Recommendations:
- Do the push-up on your knees if it is too difficult to do it fully - or "skip" it as mentioned in the "How to do it"

FLOWER

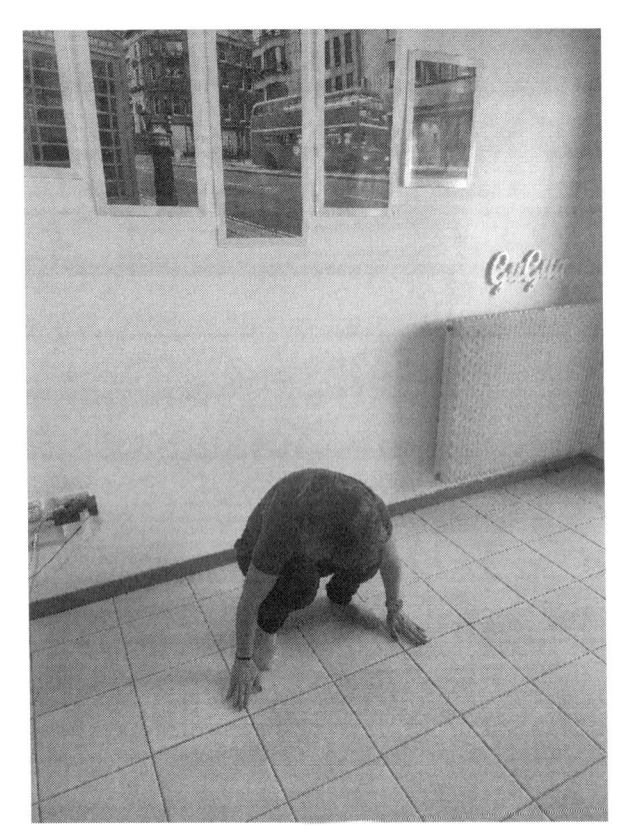

Step 1- Starting position in a deep squat with hands on the floor - inhale gently.

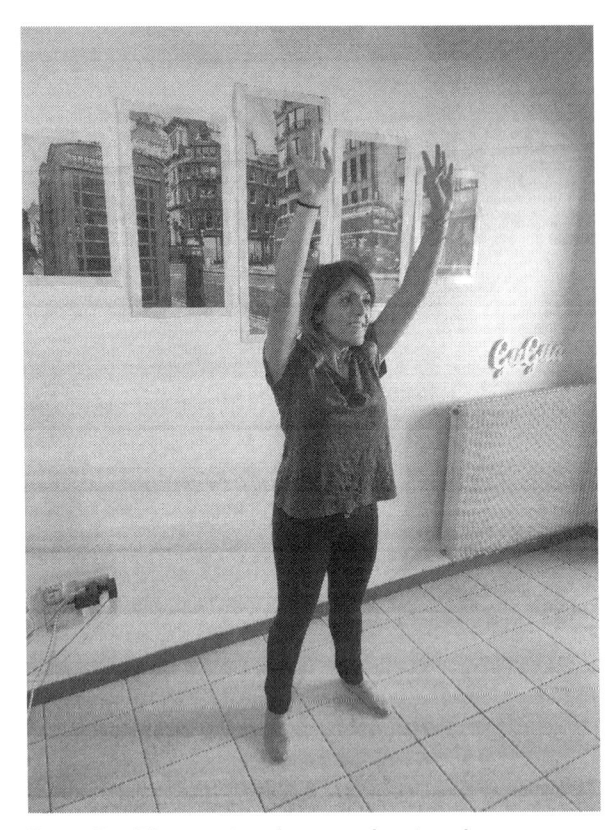

Step 2 - Then, stand up and extend your arms over your head. Exhale as you do so.

Benefits:

This exercise strengthens your lower body while working on your cardio. It is a very good exercise that aims to lose weight by burning calories. While performing the exercise it is important to keep a controlled breathing to get very present and learn to be still and surrender.

How to do it:

- Begin in a deep squat position with arms alongside the body - inhale through your nose.
- Next, stand up while extending your arms overhead, mimicking a flower blooming, and maintain the position of your feet - exhale as you stand up.
- Return to the starting position to complete one repetition.
- Repeat the exercise for the mentioned reps.

OPEN UP PLANK

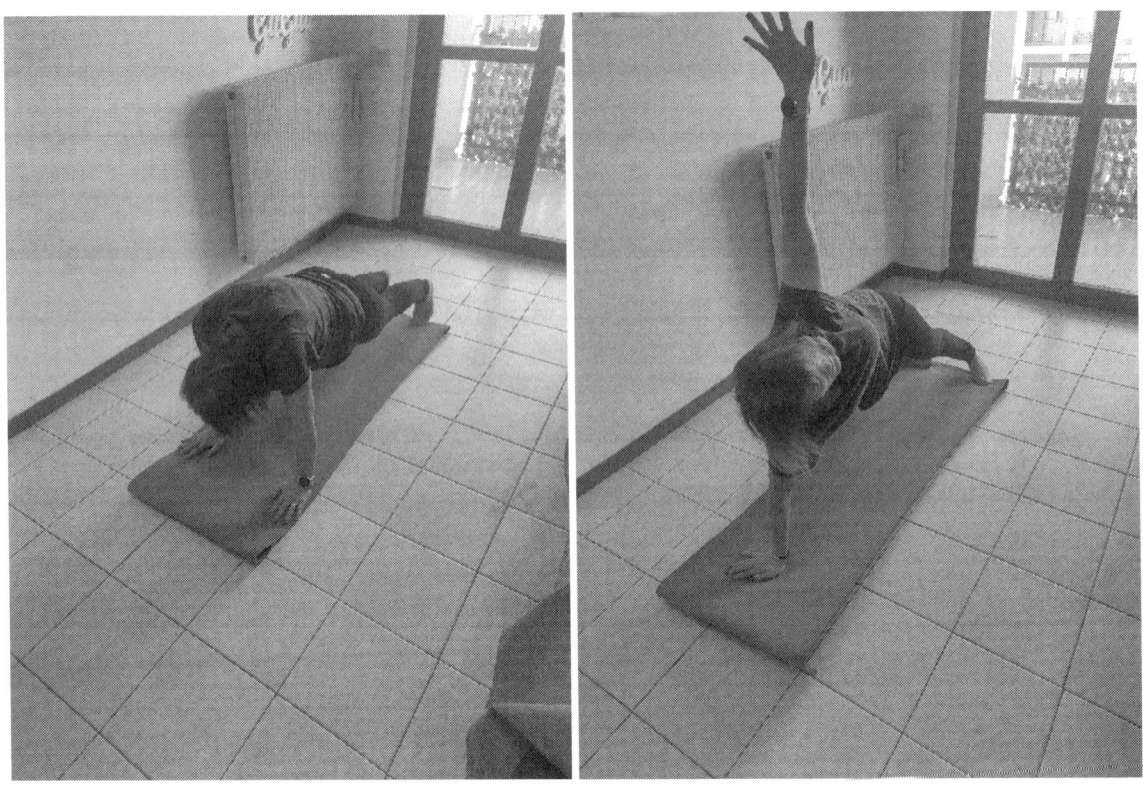

Step 1 - Starting Position with arms straight and body in a straight line.

Step 2 - Rotate towards the side and extend your arm towards the ceiling. Then, come back into the starting position.

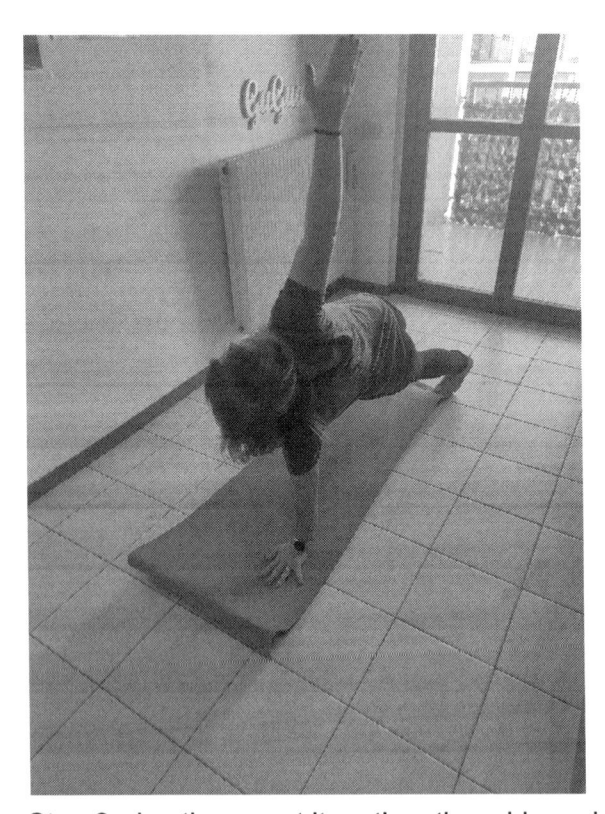

Step 3 - Lastly, repeat it on the other side and keep alternating the reps..

Benefits:

This exercise is fantastic for strengthening the core and harmonizing the entire body. It qualifies as a full-body workout because it engages various muscles simultaneously.

How to do it:

- Start in a push up position with your arms below your shoulders and feet close to each other - Body in a straight line, as shown in the first image.
- From there, open up your body towards the left side, and extend your left arm towards the ceiling - exhale as you do so.
- Hold the position for 1 second. Then, come back into the starting position.
- Then, repeat it for the mentioned reps. Lastly, repeat on the other side.

28-DAY PLAN

This 28-day plan is a great way to improve your mental and physical health. Just a few minutes a day doing specific exercises can bring a big change.

This plan does more than just give you exercises; it also helps you better understand your body and emotions. You will not only become more flexible and strong, but you will also learn to cope better with stress and anxiety.

This practice connects your body and mind by using simple breathing techniques to relax tight muscles and calm your mind. During exercises, focusing on your breath allows you to be more 'in the moment.'

Breathing and body awareness have immense influence. This programme will not only make you feel better, but it is also going to make you look better. Less stress results in a more fresh, relaxed appearance.

The most common feedback received about the plan are:

- **"Helped me with my anxiety"**
  As explained in the introduction, the difference between this practice and others like yoga and Pilates is the fact that somatic exercise is more of a sensory experience. It allows you to release negative emotions and more easily create positive ones.

- **"Feeling more flexible and reduce back pain"**
  The exercises offer various physical benefits. You'll quickly notice that increased flexibility is one of the changes you'll experience, even after just a couple of sessions."

- **"I wake up looking forward to do these exercises"**
  Many people wake up each morning without excitement for their day ahead. However, these exercises can instantly evoke a 'feel-good' sensation, motivating you to eagerly wake up and engage in them.

- **"It reduced my stress"**
The exercises aim to release tightness in the muscles, which is linked to stress. Moreover, the incorporated breathing patterns naturally help reduce stress levels. Maintaining consistency will significantly boost your results.

- **"It is the best moment of the day, I feel present"** Concentrating on deep breathing during these exercises naturally brings a sense of presence, creating a very enjoyable experience. The more you practice, the better you'll become at achieving this state.

- **"I have been told by several colleagues I look younger after doing these exercises"**
You'll not just feel better but also look better. Stress, anxiety, and trauma can age us faster, but Somatic exercises act as their antidote.

Important note! Before every session perform the exercise: *Floor Star* (Pag. 9).

DAY 1 - Repeat twice

EXERCISE	REPETITIONS	PAGE NUMBER
BABY STRETCH	4 reps	11
CHEST OPENING	3 reps each side	21
ENERGY OPENING	4 reps	51
STANDING SPIDER	4 reps each side (alternated)	45
EAGLE POSE	4 reps each side	15
REACH BACK	4 reps each side (alternated)	35
JUMPING JACKS	20 seconds	59

DAY 2 - Repeat twice

EXERCISE	REPETITIONS	PAGE NUMBER
PELVIC PREPARATION	4 reps	13
SPINAL WAVE	6 reps	33
STAR GLUTE BRIDGE	5 reps	41
OPEN LIFE	5 reps	57
NECK RELEASE	4 reps each side (alternated)	55
STANDING STRESS RELEASE	3 reps	43
STANDING REACH	4 reps	37

DAY 3 - Repeat twice

EXERCISE	REPETITIONS	PAGE NUMBER
FULL BODY ROCKING	20 seconds	47
SUPERMAN	5 reps each side	29
SPIDER CIRCLE	6 reps	39
SIDE REACH	5 each side	31
KNEE HOLD	4 each side (alternated)	53
CHEST OPENING	3 reps each side	21
FLOWER	4 reps	63

DAY 4 - Repeat twice

EXERCISE	REPETITIONS	PAGE NUMBER
FULL BODY ROCKING	20 seconds	47
NECK AND HIPS	6 reps each side	19
OPEN LIFE	5 reps	57
MOVING ROCK	20 seconds	17
STRETCH AND COMPRESS	3 reps each side (alternated)	49
REACH BACK	4 reps each side (alternated)	35
BABY STRETCH	4 reps	11

DAY 5 - Repeat twice

EXERCISE	REPETITIONS	PAGE NUMBER
ROLL IN	4 reps	25
ROLL OUT	4 reps	27
DESPAIR	4 reps	23
STANDING SPIDER	4 reps each side (alternated)	45
BURPEES	20 seconds	61
NECK RELEASE	4 reps each side (alternated)	55
SIDE REACH	5 each side	31
STANDING STRESS RELEASE	3 reps	43

DAY 6 - Repeat twice

EXERCISE	REPETITIONS	PAGE NUMBER
ENERGY OPENING	5 reps	51
EAGLE POSE	4 reps each side	15
SUPERMAN	5 reps each side	29
OPEN UP PLANK	4 reps each side	65
SPINAL WAVE	6 reps	33
STAR GLUTE BRIDGE	5 reps	41
STANDING REACH	4 reps	37
MOVING ROCK	20 seconds	17

DAY 7 - Repeat only once

EXERCISE	REPETITIONS	PAGE NUMBER
SPIDER CIRCLE	6 reps	39
KNEE HOLD	4 each side (alternated)	53
NECK AND HIPS	6 reps each side	19
DESPAIR	5 reps	23
STRETCH AND COMPRESS	3 reps each side (alternated)	49
REACH BACK	4 reps each side (alternated)	35
PELVIC PREPARATION	4 reps	13

DAY 8 - Repeat three times

EXERCISE	REPETITIONS	PAGE NUMBER
BABY STRETCH	4 reps	11
CHEST OPENING	4 reps each side	21
ENERGY OPENING	4 reps	51
STANDING SPIDER	4 reps each side (alternated)	45
EAGLE POSE	5 reps each side	15
REACH BACK	5 reps each side (alternated)	35

DAY 9 - Repeat three times

EXERCISE	REPETITIONS	PAGE NUMBER
PELVIC PREPARATION	5 reps	13
SPINAL WAVE	8 reps	33
STAR GLUTE BRIDGE	5 reps	41
OPEN LIFE	6 reps	57
NECK RELEASE	4 reps each side (alternated)	55
STANDING STRESS RELEASE	3 reps	43
STANDING REACH	6 reps	37

DAY 10 - Repeat three times

EXERCISE	REPETITIONS	PAGE NUMBER
FULL BODY ROCKING	30 seconds	47
SUPERMAN	6 reps each side	29
SPIDER CIRCLE	8 reps	39
BURPEES	20 seconds	61
SIDE REACH	5 each side	31
KNEE HOLD	6 each side (alternated)	53
CHEST OPENING	3 reps each side	21

DAY 11 - Repeat three times

EXERCISE	REPETITIONS	PAGE NUMBER
FULL BODY ROCKING	20 seconds	47
NECK AND HIPS	6 reps each side	19
OPEN LIFE	6 reps	57
MOVING ROCK	30 seconds	17
STRETCH AND COMPRESS	4 reps each side (alternated)	49
REACH BACK	4 reps each side (alternated)	35
BABY STRETCH	5 reps	11

DAY 12 - Repeat three times

EXERCISE	REPETITIONS	PAGE NUMBER
ROLL IN	4 reps	25
ROLL OUT	4 reps	27
DESPAIR	5 reps	23
STANDING SPIDER	6 reps each side (alternated)	45
NECK RELEASE	5 reps each side (alternated)	55
SIDE REACH	5 each side	31
STANDING STRESS RELEASE	4 reps	43

DAY 13 - Repeat three times

EXERCISE	REPETITIONS	PAGE NUMBER
ENERGY OPENING	6 reps	51
EAGLE POSE	4 reps each side	15
SUPERMAN	5 reps each side	29
SPINAL WAVE	8 reps	33
OPEN UP PLANK	5 reps each side	65
STAR GLUTE BRIDGE	6 reps	41
STANDING REACH	5 reps	37
MOVING ROCK	30 seconds	17

DAY 14 - Repeat once

EXERCISE	REPETITIONS	PAGE NUMBER
SPIDER CIRCLE	8 reps	39
KNEE HOLD	4 reps each side (alternated)	53
NECK AND HIPS	6 reps each side	19
DESPAIR	5 reps	23
STRETCH AND COMPRESS	4 reps each side (alternated)	49
REACH BACK	4 reps each side (alternated)	35
PELVIC PREPARATION	4 reps	13

DAY 15 - Repeat four times

EXERCISE	REPETITIONS	PAGE NUMBER
BABY STRETCH	4 reps	11
CHEST OPENING	5 reps each side	21
ENERGY OPENING	4 reps	51
STANDING SPIDER	5 reps each side (alternated)	45
EAGLE POSE	5 reps each side	15
REACH BACK	5 reps each side (alternated)	35
JUMPING JACKS	30 seconds	59

DAY 16 - Repeat four times

EXERCISE	REPETITIONS	PAGE NUMBER
PELVIC PREPARATION	5 reps	13
SPINAL WAVE	8 reps	33
STAR GLUTE BRIDGE	7 reps	41
OPEN LIFE	6 reps	57
NECK RELEASE	4 reps each side (alternated)	55
STANDING STRESS RELEASE	5 reps	43
STANDING REACH	6 reps	37

DAY 17 - Repeat four times

EXERCISE	REPETITIONS	PAGE NUMBER
FULL BODY ROCKING	30 seconds	47
SUPERMAN	6 reps each side	29
FLOWER	5 reps	63
SPIDER CIRCLE	8 reps	39
SIDE REACH	5 each side	31
KNEE HOLD	6 each side (alternated)	53
CHEST OPENING	5 reps each side	21

DAY 18 - Repeat four times

EXERCISE	REPETITIONS	PAGE NUMBER
FULL BODY ROCKING	20 seconds	47
NECK AND HIPS	7 reps each side	19
OPEN LIFE	6 reps	57
MOVING ROCK	30 seconds	17
STRETCH AND COMPRESS	5 reps each side (alternated)	49
REACH BACK	5 reps each side (alternated)	35
BABY STRETCH	6 reps	11

DAY 19 - Repeat four times

EXERCISE	REPETITIONS	PAGE NUMBER
ROLL IN	5 reps	25
ROLL OUT	5 reps	27
DESPAIR	6 reps	23
STANDING SPIDER	6 reps each side (alternated)	45
NECK RELEASE	6 reps each side (alternated)	55
SIDE REACH	6 each side	31
STANDING STRESS RELEASE	5 reps	43

DAY 20 - Repeat four times

EXERCISE	REPETITIONS	PAGE NUMBER
ENERGY OPENING	6 reps	51
EAGLE POSE	6 reps each side	15
SUPERMAN	6 reps each side	29
SPINAL WAVE	8 reps	33
STAR GLUTE BRIDGE	8 reps	41
STANDING REACH	7 reps	37
MOVING ROCK	30 seconds	17

DAY 21 - Repeat once

EXERCISE	REPETITIONS	PAGE NUMBER
SPIDER CIRCLE	10 reps	39
KNEE HOLD	6 reps each side (alternated)	53
FLOWER	6 reps	63
NECK AND HIPS	8 reps each side	19
DESPAIR	5 reps	23
STRETCH AND COMPRESS	6 reps each side (alternated)	49
REACH BACK	6 reps each side (alternated)	35
PELVIC PREPARATION	4 reps	13

DAY 22 - Repeat four times

EXERCISE	REPETITIONS	PAGE NUMBER
BABY STRETCH	6 reps	11
CHEST OPENING	5 reps each side	21
BURPEES	30 seconds	61
ENERGY OPENING	6 reps	51
STANDING SPIDER	6 reps each side (alternated)	45
EAGLE POSE	5 reps each side	15
REACH BACK	5 reps each side (alternated)	35

DAY 23 - Repeat four times

EXERCISE	REPETITIONS	PAGE NUMBER
PELVIC PREPARATION	6 reps	13
SPINAL WAVE	8 reps	33
STAR GLUTE BRIDGE	7 reps	41
OPEN LIFE	8 reps	57
NECK RELEASE	5 reps each side (alternated)	55
STANDING STRESS RELEASE	6 reps	43
STANDING REACH	6 reps	37

DAY 24 - Repeat four times

EXERCISE	REPETITIONS	PAGE NUMBER
FULL BODY ROCKING	45 seconds	47
SUPERMAN	6 reps each side	29
SPIDER CIRCLE	10 reps	39
SIDE REACH	6 each side	31
KNEE HOLD	6 each side (alternated)	53
CHEST OPENING	7 reps each side	21

DAY 25 - Repeat four times

EXERCISE	REPETITIONS	PAGE NUMBER
FULL BODY ROCKING	30 seconds	47
NECK AND HIPS	7 reps each side	19
OPEN LIFE	8 reps	57
MOVING ROCK	45 seconds	17
STRETCH AND COMPRESS	6 reps each side (alternated)	49
REACH BACK	7 reps each side (alternated)	35
BABY STRETCH	7 reps	11

DAY 26 - Repeat four times

EXERCISE	REPETITIONS	PAGE NUMBER
ROLL IN	7 reps	25
ROLL OUT	7 reps	27
DESPAIR	6 reps	23
OPEN UP PLANK	6 reps each side	65
STANDING SPIDER	8 reps each side (alternated)	45
NECK RELEASE	6 reps each side (alternated)	55
SIDE REACH	7 each side	31
STANDING STRESS RELEASE	6 reps	43

DAY 27 - Repeat four times

EXERCISE	REPETITIONS	PAGE NUMBER
ENERGY OPENING	8 reps	51
EAGLE POSE	8 reps each side	15
SUPERMAN	7 reps each side	29
SPINAL WAVE	10 reps	33
STAR GLUTE BRIDGE	8 reps	41
STANDING REACH	8 reps	37
MOVING ROCK	45 seconds	17

DAY 28 - Repeat once

EXERCISE	REPETITIONS	PAGE NUMBER
SPIDER CIRCLE	12 reps	39
KNEE HOLD	8 reps each side (alternated)	53
NECK AND HIPS	8 reps each side	19
DESPAIR	5 reps	23
STRETCH AND COMPRESS	6 reps each side (alternated)	49
REACH BACK	8 reps each side (alternated)	35
PELVIC PREPARATION	4 reps	13
JUMPING JACKS	30 seconds	59

CONCLUSION

Well done! You've finished learning about somatic exercises and their incredible benefits. These exercises benefit both your body and mind.

You've discovered that these exercises are about more than just moving. They assist you in relaxing, reducing stress, and feeling more connected to yourself. The 28-day plan functions as a road map. You will undoubtedly notice changes if you stick to it and perform the exercises on a regular basis.

However, keep in mind that this is not the end. Continue with these exercises while paying attention to your body's sensations. Apply the positive emotions you felt during these exercises into your daily life.

As mentioned at the beginning of the book, **for any questions or doubts related to somatic training and exercises feel free to email me at** mertoncoreyfitness@gmail.com - Looking forward to hearing from you!

I hope these exercises continue to make you feel good and strong. Thank you for joining me on this journey to better health. Now keep going and strive to be the best you can be!

Printed in Great Britain
by Amazon